1984

# The Complete Hospice Guide

By the same author

*First American Hospice: Three Years of Home Care*
(with Sylvia Lack, M.D.)

*A Special Kind of Love: Care for the Dying Child*

# The Complete Hospice Guide

by Robert W. Buckingham

1817

HARPER & ROW, PUBLISHERS, New York
Cambridge, Philadelphia, San Francisco
London, Mexico City, São Paulo, Sydney

*For My Father*

Grateful acknowledgment is made for permission to reprint the poem on page 121, from *The Complete Poems of Emily Dickinson*, edited by Thomas H. Johnson. Copyright 1929 by Martha Dickinson Bianchi; copyright © renewed 1957 by Mary L. Hampson.

FIRST EDITION

*Designer: C. Linda Dingler*

Library of Congress Cataloging in Publication Data

Buckingham, Robert W.
    The complete hospice guide.

    Includes index.
    1. Terminal care.    2. Terminal care—United States.
3. Terminal care facilities—United States—
Directories.    I. Title.
R726.8.B8    1983        362.1′75        83-47527
ISBN 0-06-015192-7              83 84 85 86 87 10 9 8 7 6 5 4 3 2 1
ISBN 0-06-091084-4 (pbk.)       83 84 85 86 87 10 9 8 7 6 5 4 3 2 1

# Contents

# Acknowledgments

I wish to acknowledge the wonders of four special women. Leah Loveday has been an inspiration to my work. She was always there when I needed her help. Her comments, editing, and research have made this book possible. Dr. Sylvia Lack, former medical director of the first hospice in the United States, has given me knowledge and understanding of the philosophy and practice of hospice care. She is truly the leader of the hospice movement in the United States and is responsible for many excellent programs in this country. Sallie Coolidge, my editor at Harper & Row, has been an ideal guide and has shaped this book with her sensitive and practical comments, suggestions, and encouragement. I am indebted to her clarity and thoroughness. And finally, let me offer my sincere appreciation to Dr. Elisabeth Kübler-Ross, the woman who motivated me and put me on this path of questioning.

# Foreword

Dying is part of the process of living. As a leaf buds and shines its youthful color, it must also mature, decay, and die. We are all temporary leaves on the tree of life. We all must fall someday. We should not fear death. We should not ignore death. We must not protect ourselves from the reality of our end. The end of our physical being should not overly concern us. We should instead be concerned about living each and every day as fully as possible.

Unfortunately, the issue of death in our society has been denied, hidden, and thus feared. The recent attempts of a few lay people have brought this important issue into people's consciousness. Many physicians, too, are strangers to the real issues of dying. Historically, physicians have been taught to diagnose, treat, and cure. They look at death as failure and therefore shy away from those dying patients whom they have "failed." More efforts must be made to educate the medical community as well as the public about the importance of hospice care.

This book attempts to familiarize the reader with the basic concepts of hospice care. Hospice is a philosophy and concept of care whose time has come. Hospice philosophy for the terminally ill incorporates pain control, symptom control (physical and psychological), continuous medical and nursing accessibility, medical direction, utilization of volunteers, home care, training of family members as care givers, and a bereavement program for the survivors.

In 1970, my fifty-year-old mother (a New York City fashion designer) was dying of cancer of the breast. She was cared for in a prestigious teaching institution. It was good general care but poor palliative care. There were no hospices then. No one talked to me, no one talked to my father or my sister. We had many questions, with no one to address them to. My mother lingered in discomfort. Death was a release for her, which I do not regret, but I regret the way she died. Many of her medical, nursing, and emotional needs were unaddressed. While traditional approaches to health care emphasize cure and the prolongation of life, such care is restrictive and insensitive to the needs of the terminal patient and the family who have accepted the reality of death and wish to focus on the quality of the life remaining.

In the early 1970s I was a graduate student in the Yale School of Medicine. Unbeknown to me at that time, an interdisciplinary faculty committee was meeting weekly at Yale, arranging to bring over from England a new concept and philosophy of medical and nursing care—hospice care. It was designed for people with a very limited prognosis (six months or less to live), and encompassed psychological, spiritual, and medical problems. Upon completion of my doctoral work at Yale, the dean of the Yale Nursing School asked if I would be interested in working as director of research at the first and only developing hospice in the country. I took the position, and it enabled me to interview and study many wonderful patients who, like my mother, were suffering from end-stage disease. These patients and their families taught me the meaning of life. I realized that through the eyes of the dying one can realize the significant issues of living.

The early days of the New Haven Hospice were very taxing to the staff. We suffered many setbacks and defeats. Educating the medical community was the most difficult task of all, and it still is. Without the support of the National Cancer Institute, the hospice concept of care in the United States would not have survived. In those years we proved to Washington and the American people that hospice care was needed in the United States. Since 1976, more than six hundred hospices have developed nationwide. I am happy to report that hospice care is now reimbursible under Medicare/ Medicaid and private insurance companies like Blue Cross and Blue Shield. We have proved that hospice care is often better than traditional acute-care facilities and considerably less expensive.

Historically—since the industrial revolution—dying has been a coming-apart experience for most families. Hospice care concentrates on making the process of dying a *coming-together* experience for patient and family. Hospice is not a place or an institution but a philosophy of care in which the person is considered of primary importance and the disease is secondary. For the last ten years, I have spent my academic career developing, managing, researching, and teaching about the hospice concept of care. It is my lifelong wish to have the word "hospice" disappear and the concept and philosophy of hospice care prevail with all medical, nursing, and allied health professionals.

My ten years of research into the hospice concept have brought me to the belief that in order to live the way you choose, you must be assertive. That applies to how you die, as well. Many people are more content to be regulated by others than to take charge of their own lives. Epictetus wrote of freedom in his *Discourses*: "No man is free who is not master of himself." Freedom to choose the way we live and die is what families and patients must strive for.

I hope this book will help to show readers the way to live as fully as possible.

*Tucson, Arizona*
*April 1983*

This book is based on my experiences with hospice care. The names I have used are not real names, and I have altered the details of locales and individual case histories where necessary.

# Introduction

Hospice is a concept of medical, nursing, and spiritual care, an attitude toward death and the care of the dying. It is a way of dying. Terminal disease is managed so that patients can live comfortably until they die, cared for by family and friends. And families, bereaved, are sustained by hospice.

Dying is not only a physical process; it is a psychological and an emotional process, a spiritual and a social process. The process of dying is part of the process of living. We should not deny it. American perspectives on death and dying seem to me strangely paradoxical. Our news media confront the fact of death directly, whether with oversize headlines or with unobtrusive statements on the obituary page. At the same time, speaking about death and dying has been a taboo topic in our culture, though the work and the writing of Elisabeth Kübler-Ross have done much to break this taboo. It has been taboo because it has been hidden. Certainly, we Americans hesitate to talk openly about the process of dying. We see this fact often demonstrated by the physician who is reluctant to be totally honest with his or her patient. Physicians in this culture are trained to cure and not to care. When cure becomes impossible, their typical response is to leave the patient alone and tell the family that they have done all that medical science can do. One must understand that physicians, like the rest of us, are trained to and tempted by success. Death to them represents a failure, and failures, as we all know, are difficult to swallow.

In medical schools and hospitals, physicians and nurses may exhibit considerable skill in handling the medical mechanics of attending the dying. But rarely do they address the patient as a total person.

After ten years as a researcher with terminal cancer patients, I have found that what these people need and want most is basic relief from the indignities of their disease; continuous competent medical care; and assurance that they won't be abandoned by the medical/nursing staff and by loved ones.

The hospice concept represents a return to humanistic medicine—to care within the patient's community, family-centered care, the view of the patient as a person. The victim of a terminal illness is permitted to die with dignity. Studies indicate that the patient of a hospice program will not experience the anxiety, helplessness, inadequacy, and guilt to which a patient in an acute-care facility is prey. Furthermore, a hospice program can relieve family members and loved ones of various psychological disorders associated with loss.

Since the turn of the century, enormous alterations have taken place within American society in our attitudes toward death and dying and the role death plays in our lives. Both the age at which a person is expected to die and the place where death typically occurs have changed radically. Though people die at home, on the street, and at their place of employment, the greatest number of deaths occur in public institutions. The elderly, who so disproportionately compose our population, often die in extended-care facilities and convalescent homes. And when the aged who have been taken care of in a long-term institution begin to fail, they are frequently transported to an acute-care hospital to die.

Recently, however, there appears to be a swing back of public opinion, with a conviction that some of the problems with the care of the dying could be solved if the patient died at home, surrounded by his or her family. This feeling may be part of the "back to nature" culture, which seeks to reintegrate each human being with the life cycle. The change in attitude is also influenced by the growing realization by young and middle-aged people that we are turning into a top-heavy population. Policymakers are beginning to comprehend that they will someday be part of a population of aged for whom society as it is presently structured has no effective place. Indeed, the hospice movement can be seen as a springboard from which society's reexamination of its attitudes toward bodily deterioration, death, and decay will in turn affect our attitudes toward all unproductive members of our society: the mentally and physically handicapped, the weak, and the elderly.

This book has a twofold purpose: It is intended as a guide and introduction to the hospice concept for both interested lay people and health-care professionals. Every practical action in the world began as a thought, an idea in the hearts and minds of those who wished to improve the present situation. This book is for those concerned and compassionate individuals, whether lay or professional, who wish to explore a new alternative in the care of the dying. Before going further, it may be helpful to define hospice. The National Hospice Organization defines it as follows:

Hospice is a medically directed multidisciplinary program providing skilled care of an appropriate nature for terminally ill patients and their families to live as fully as possible until the time of death. Hospice helps relieve symptoms during the distress (physical, psychological, spiritual, social, economic) that may occur during the course of the disease, dying and bereavement.[1]

Although hospice exists as a *concept of care*, it is apparent that a distinction must be made between a hospice home-care program and a hospice inpatient facility. For those patients who do not have a family member or anyone else to act as a primary care person, and for those who need more medical care than can be offered at home, inpatient care is appropriate. Whatever environment fulfills the needs of the patient and family is the environment in which the patient should go through the dying process. As one observer has said: "The quality of the dying process is affected to a large extent by the physical surrounding in which the process occurs. The surrounding itself acts not only as a catalyst to initiate the most effective treatment for the patient as an individual but also can assist in managing the complex psychological interrelationship inextricably entwined with the patient's medical treatment."[2]

To give the patient the best possible care, basic methodologies must be established. Basically, the hospice concept asks: "What does each dying individual need? What are the needs of the family?" The needs of the patient and the family must be considered first. Home care, inpatient care, or a combination of the two may be the answer to these questions, depending upon the individual patient. A primary care person (the family member or friend who performs most of the patient's care) with hospice support generally feels more capable of meeting the patient's needs and has greater confidence in his or her ability than a primary care person without such support. Being able to take care of, provide assistance for, and give comfort to the dying patient dissipates some of the guilt and helplessness felt by the family. At the same time, when a dying patient is cared for at home, adjustments have to be made in the functioning of the family. In *First American Hospice,* Sylvia Lack and I give the foundation of the "one unit of care" concept:

Because of the disruption of family life style caused by many changes that occur during the course of terminal illness, hospice personnel recognize the importance of sustaining continuity of care. Terminal illness shatters the equilibrium of the family group; therefore it is the patient and the family who are designated as the unit of care. Medical care and supportive counseling involve both the patient and the family by day in their homes. The team is also on call for emergencies at night and weekends.[3]

Effective hospice care means that patient and family are treated together as one unit. Problems of the patient and the family are inevitably intertwined. It is virtually impossible for family members providing care to a dying patient to camouflage their feelings; at the same time, the patient will (and should) display his feelings openly. For this to remain a productive interchange, hospice staff is necessary for support. *First American Hospice* states:

> Patients' behavioral patterns often undergo a marked change, and overlapping defenses of denial and symptoms of depression dominate their relationships with others. At this time the medical personnel, and more especially the families, desperately need to understand that the patient's changed behavior is not a result of something they may or may not have done but a predictable response to a very difficult situation. Only when feelings of anger, guilt, and loneliness experienced by the family members are vented and dissipated can the unspoken sense of alienation in the dying patient be alleviated. Family problems are often too closely related to interaction with the terminally ill cancer patient to go unheeded.[4]

The point is made continually in the literature on hospice care that patient and family should not be separated. The patient needs to be listened to, cared for, and supported. The same applies to the family, with an added emphasis on educating them to understand the course of the disease. The better informed family members are, the less anxiety exists. An important task of hospice workers is to find out what the family's life style was like before terminal illness. The emphasis is on the well-being of the patient and the family, with all their individual preferences and varieties of life style. Hospice care adapts to meet these varied individual needs, rather than adapting patient and family to an institutional program. Patient and family are active in this process and shape the care that is offered. Teaching and supporting each other, they share with the staff the experience of dying. Family and staff cooperate in caring for the patient, and later give and receive support in bereavement.

Medical, governmental, and educational institutions have recognized the profound urgency for the advocacy of the hospice concept. As a result, a considerable change in policy and attitude has occurred in the last ten years. As the hospice movement grows, it does more than alter our treatment of the dying. Hospices and home care are de-escalating the soaring costs of illness by reducing the individual and collective burdens borne by all health insurance policyholders. Because hospice and home care use no sophisticated diagnostic treatment, their overhead is basically for personal care and medication. The cost of a hospice stay is projected to be significantly less than that of the hospital stay. At present, health insurance programs are not geared to cope with hospice techniques and will not reimburse their services. Ironically, getting a patient out of bed and out of his home usually disrupts his coverage. Hospice, Inc., in Branford, Connecticut, the first American hospice, has made formal recommendations that Medicare be extended to cover anyone of any age with a limited life prognosis.

In his book *Dying,* John Hinton says that "the emphasis must always lie upon tending the person, not battling with his disease, treating the one who feels symptoms, not just treating the symptoms."[5] And in *The Hospice Movement,* Sandol Stoddard speaks of hospice as a "caring community," coexisting with a belief that the patient is something more than his body.[6] The dying patient must not be abandoned or isolated from his usual sources of spiritual and emotional support; he needs to know that he matters as a *human being* to those around him at this time. This holistic approach to caring for the dying is a concept that pervades the current literature on the subject.

The primary message that must be conveyed to the dying patient is that he is unique, and that his needs are special and will be met in an individual way. Although standard reactions to the knowledge of imminent death may be experienced and expressed, we must not lose sight of the meaning these feelings hold for the dying individual within the unique pattern of a life no other person has lived and within a particular environment, while he suffers from a particular disease syndrome. What is distinctive about this person's life may be more significant than the universal situation he has in common with many others. Cicely Saunders says so well what should be said to all dying patients: "You matter because you are you. You matter to the last moment of your life, and we will do all we can not only to help you die peacefully, but also to live until you die."[7] Cicely Saunders's method of helping patients live until they die is accomplished through effective pain and symptom control. The first step in alleviating uncomfortable symptoms and easing pain is to listen to the patient, who alone can best describe the suffering. Once the symptoms and the nature of the pain have been identified, appropriate measures can be taken to alleviate it. "Pain control it turns out is not so much a matter of what it is in the medicine, as it is of how and when it is administered."[8]

So much of chronic pain in cancer patients is perpetuated by "PRN," letters which stand for the Latin phrase *pro re nata*—"whenever necessary." This prescription, used by physicians, dictates that the patient be given medication at the onset of pain. The problem lies precisely here, for medication should instead be given *prior to* the onset of pain. "The fear of pain increases pain itself by geometric proportions. When severe pain is experienced and is expected to continue indefinitely or even to get worse, the patient enters a world of horror and hopelessness that for many treated by conventional methods ends only with death. This is not necessary and with hospice care it simply does not happen. Knowing that it does not happen is, in itself, part of the comfort offered to hospice patients and families.[9] The administration of medication whenever necessary fosters dependency on medication. When medication is not administered until the onset of pain, the patient must experience pain while waiting for medication, and continue to experience it while waiting for it to take effect; then the process begins again while the next onset is anticipated. Dying patients feel enough loss without having to sacrifice more of their independence and limited time.

It is for these very reasons that the alleviation of symptoms and the control of chronic pain are of primary importance in terminal care. Hospice staffs have become knowledgeable about the management of symptoms and pain. Freed from deep suffering, the patient has more time and energy to respond to family and friends. With a mind unoccupied with the anticipation and experience of pain, the patient can put his "house in order." Family and staff also feel relief and are more comfortable along with the patient. Obviously, pain management is a high priority. In the process of dying, it is extremely important that the relationships between patient and family are lived out and concluded as productively as possible. In many ways, dying is a "bringing together" process. Unfortunately, this is not fostered when the patient is dying in an acute-care hospital or a long-term-care nursing home. Restricted visiting hours, institutional rules, the alien and unhomelike environment tend to inhibit family participation in caring for the patient. Hospice, whether home or inpatient, serves the whole family as the unit of care, and involves the family in the patient's care. The patient does not become foreign to his own family, and communication and unity are facilitated. Families are drawn together and loved ones can give each other the support they need. "A family's active participation in care is also part of the separation process itself, which includes giving and receiving, coming together and letting go."[10]

Throughout discussion of the needs of the dying patient, it appears that the patient does all the receiving—is treated as a unique individual, has symptoms alleviated, pain controlled, and people given access. Yet it is of vital importance to realize that the dying are just as involved in giving as in receiving. We who care for the dying must be aware of this; we must allow this process to occur. "With the spread of the hospice in our culture, many of us discover that we are learning from the sick how to be well again and from the dying how to live."[11]

Hospice concepts today provide a catalyst for change in our attitudes toward the care of the dying. For the last few decades, our society has ignored the plight of the dying in our desire to deny the inevitability of death. In our compulsion to prolong life at any cost, we have developed technological apparatus to sustain the body. Death, in this view, is not a natural event but a technological failure. Our definition of life becomes narrow (and meaningless) if it signifies biological continuance only. In our desire to extend physical life we have needlessly prolonged the suffering of dying individuals. We have mismedicated, leaving patients in distress and discomfort, surrounded by apparatus and routines rather than family and friends. The survivors have been nearly as lonely and isolated, without the peace and satisfaction of caring for someone they love.

Hospice concepts of care are not concerned with prolonging life when cure is no longer a possibility, but focus on the quality of life. The total being is sustained—psychologically, physically, and spiritually. Symptom control is emphasized not only for the patient's comfort but also so that he may be free to work out the spiritual and emotional aspects of dying. His life's meaning may become more apparent as he takes the time to review it, and as he gives and shares love. The gifts of the dying can be precious, for as social masks slip away, the dying are often able to communicate on a deeper level with those around them. It is extremely valuable for the living to see life from a different perspective, to experience it from a more timeless vantage point. Those who have witnessed a peaceful death are less fearful of their own life's end, and accept death more naturally. There is much we can learn about life from the dying; thus that basic hospice concept of the patient as giver as well as receiver.

It is exciting to see the eagerness with which hospices have been greeted in this country. Popular enthusiasm has been coupled with careful planning and the reeducation of medical personnel and lay people. Hospice is an idea whose time has come. People are relearning what the ancients always told us, that death is a natural part of life. The hospice movement itself is helping to reshape medical and nursing attitudes, for as more doctors and nurses come in contact with it, more are educated by its holistic concepts.

Working with the dying need not be morbid or depressing, but can reaffirm our humanity. Also, as we accept nature's ecology, it is hoped that we will not prolong life meaninglessly, but conclude, with Cicely Saunders, that sometimes dying is the healthy thing to do.[12]

# 1 ❧
# Hospice History and Philosophy

## History

Hospitality, hospitable, host, hostess, hospital, hostel, hotel, hospice—all these words have the same root. All include the ideas of kindness and generosity to strangers, or caring for our fellow beings and offering them nourishment and refreshment.

Ancient hospices or hospitals (for the two were one for a number of centuries) were a sanctuary for the poor wayfarer, the sick and dying, the woman in labor, the orphan, the needy, and the religious pilgrim. Medieval hospices were generally run by religious orders and served the Lord in serving His poor, His sick, and those in need of shelter. Welcome was extended in hospices throughout Europe, in major towns and cities, in villages, in remote monastic hermitages, and along the route to the Holy Land. Hospices offered refuge as long as two thousand years ago. The Knights of Hospitallers of the Order of St. John of Jerusalem in the twelfth century A.D. offered aid to pilgrims and the sick throughout Europe, and at one time were active and held land in Rhodes, Cyprus, Italy, Germany, and England. If hospice workers were unkind to patients, or neglected them in any way, they ate bread and water for a week and were whipped.[1] The records of the Knights Hospitallers, kept for six hundred years, show their efforts to maintain their ideals and goals, despite increasing wealth and land holdings. At their hospice, or hospital, in Rhodes, the incurably ill, sheltered in a group of rooms reserved for travelers and pilgrims, were cared for apart from those with other illnesses.

In the medieval view, life was not separate from dying, for all who lived must die. Pilgrims, travelers, and the dying were therefore housed together, for all were on a journey and needed a place to stop for comfort. The news the travelers brought was of value to the medieval stay-at-home, and the dying were also valued as individuals and as beings whose existence was moving on to a higher plane.

Monasteries were closed in many countries during the Reformation, and gradually the concepts of hospice and hospital became separate. Today, the responsibility of caring for the sick and dying, formerly private or religious, has become a public, or government, function.[2] Science has supported medicine with marvelous discoveries to cure disease and prolong life, but the modern hospital increasingly has the look and feel of a laboratory. The bureaucracy needed to support the hospital system creates demands upon the time and energy of medical staff and patients as well. The modern hospital is well equipped to aid in an acute, life-threatening situation, but it is seldom equipped to offer comfort to a traveler near his journey's end. Now, after a lapse of several centuries, hospices are again caring for the dying and their families, due in large part to the work of Cicely Saunders in England and Elisabeth Kübler-Ross in the United States.

In the late 1940s, Dr. Saunders became friends with a man in his forties dying of cancer in a busy London hospital. As they talked, the ideas of a place that could meet the needs of the dying—which could have met his needs—grew. Together they shared a dream of a haven where others like him could die in peace and dignity. This man, who had escaped from the Warsaw ghetto, died in 1948, leaving £500 to Dr. Saunders, and saying, "I'll be a window in your Home."[3]

St. Christopher's Hospice grew from this gift, and from the work and planning of other donors over the next decade. The name "hospice" had been revived by the Irish Sisters of Chai..., who began opening homes for dying patients in the nineteenth century. St. Christopher's was planned to combine the old concept of hospitality and care with the modern skills of a hospital.

Inaugurated with nearly all the funds needed for land, building, and equipment, St. Christopher's has continued to expand its services, including a Domiciliary Service Program, which educates staff and students and visitors, and it is the model from which other hospices have grown both in England and in the United States. Financial needs are partially met by contracts with the National Health Service, with the deficits made up by gifts. True to the old hospice ideal, no patient is refused services because of inability to pay. "Giving care is St. Christopher's only way of fund raising."[4]

Patients are admitted to the hospice at their doctors' request. They come with various diseases with a terminal prognosis, some to stay and others to return home again, and a few who have improved return to a treatment hospital. Whatever the disease or the prognosis, all patients receive personal care and are greeted by name upon admission and throughout their stay. Bereaved families are supported by visits from St. Christopher's staff and volunteers. Relatives of deceased patients are remembered with anniversary cards the first year after bereavement, and are welcome to services at the chapel, to a monthly social club, and to general parties to which staff and their families are also invited. Like residents of a small village, St. Christopher's staff, patients, and families have a feeling of community, a family feeling.

Dr. Saunders visited Yale in the early 1960s and spoke of her efforts on behalf of the terminally ill. By the time St. Christopher's was serving patients, a group of clergymen and medical people in New Haven were making efforts to develop an American hospice. Florence Wald, R.N., former dean of the Yale University School of Nursing, investigated the need for hospice in New Haven. Reverend Edward Dobihal, clinical professor of pastoral care at Yale Divinity School and director of religious ministries at the Yale–New Haven Hospital, had long been concerned about the care of the terminally ill in his ministry and was a contributor to the study, which was finished in late 1969. The next few years saw incorporation, the formulation of a hospice philosophy, and a donation which enabled Hospice of New Haven to rent a small office and to hire Florence Wald and three others. Later, Dr. Sylvia Lack of St. Christopher's was hired as the first medical director.

Progress was slow, and when local opposition prohibited land purchase for a facility, the founders realized that they needed to prepare and educate the public to receive hospice. Some neighborhoods feared having a "death house" nearby. Beginning in mid-1974, patients were being served by the home-care program, and by fall 1974, funds were received from the National Cancer Institute and the Kaiser Foundation. A receptive community was found by late 1976.

The New Haven hospice was the first of three demonstration projects funded by the National Cancer Institute; the others were in Boonton, New Jersey, and Tucson, Arizona. Two fundamental difficulties were faced; first, the status quo for terminal care in the American medical community; and second, the need to fit hospice services into the bureaucracy of contemporary health care without compromising ideals and goals. Many in the medical establishment expressed doubts at first, and thought hospice, and palliative home care particularly, would be unacceptable in this country. Planners were told "when Americans are sick, they want to be in a hospital. Nobody dies at home in this country; the society isn't set up for it."[5]

The response of patients and families proved otherwise: A service emphasizing care rather than technology can be accepted by both lay people and professionals. Evaluation studies done at the time (1974–1976, during which I was hospice director of research) show that hospice services benefit patients and families and that these benefits are measurable. For example, in a quasi-experimental control study I conducted for my dissertation for the Yale School of Medicine, I found that primary care persons with hospice support showed less anxiety and hostility than primary care persons without such support. Hospice, Inc., New Haven, and the

National Cancer Institute have demonstrated that many people in this country do desire home care and are willing to make sacrifices and adjustments in order to keep a family member at home.

Since Hospice Inc., New Haven, began serving patients in 1974, the concept has spread rapidly. Communities throughout the country have sought hospice services and are creating facilities. The National Hospice Organization (NHO) 1980 directory lists 138 member organizations providing service,[6] but present estimates run as high as 500 for hospices in varying stages of development.

Hospice is a flexible concept which can fit into many settings. Some hospices are functioning today with a base in an established hospital; others have independent inpatient facilities, or affiliations with another community service. Not all American hospices offer inpatient care, but home care and bereavement programs seem to be the norm. It appears that two divergent types of hospices are developing: (1) independent, heavily volunteer hospices with unstable funding, in which a variety of professional staff deliver a wide array of social/psychological services; and (2) institutionally based hospices providing both inpatient and home care, supplying a greater variety of medical/nursing services but fewer social/psychological services, using a smaller number of volunteers and paid staff, and experiencing no funding problems. A recent study which I undertook with Dale Lupu indicates that the funding mix varies considerably from program to program. Private sources (individuals and foundations) provided support to a majority of hospices; third-party payers (private carriers, Medicare, Medicaid, state and local government) are also prevalent, despite the lack of any specific national public programs to reimburse such services as: physician home visits, pastoral care, volunteer directors, homemakers, and education.

Yet in spite of some funding difficulties, the hospice concept is well and thriving in the eighties. Congress recently voted to extend Medicare coverage to hospice care (mainly because it is less expensive than hospitals or nursing homes). Though such coverage is limited, it indicates national recognition of the value of the hospice by a wide variety of people. In less than a decade since the first hospice patients were cared for in New Haven, the concept has achieved such recognition that Ronald Reagan declared November 7–14, 1982, as National Hospice Week to encourage government agencies, the medical community, private organizations, and citizens to participate in programs to encourage "national recognition and support for the hospice care concept." The hospice idea is springing up and taking root in our time, as in ages past. Hospices are also flourishing in Canada, Japan, Italy, Denmark, and Sweden.

## Philosophy of Care

Hospice is a humane and sensible approach to terminal illness, combining care, comfort, and the support of family and friends as the individual faces death. The following principles constitute appropriate care for the dying and their families.*

- The patient needs to be as symptom-free as possible so that his energy can be used to live the remaining portion of his life as fully as possible.
- Doctors and nurses must be easily accessible to the patient and to family members.
- Continuity of care should be sustained by the same health team, regardless of whether the patient is in the hospital or at home.
- The patient's and the family's life style must be maintained and their life philosophies respected by the professional health-care givers.
- Loneliness, isolation, and fears of abandonment are significant sources of anguish to patients who are dying. Professional and lay health-care givers must be prepared to address the problem when it surfaces.
- Twenty-four-hour care must be available to the patient and to family members.
- No one person can fully meet the needs of the dying. A multidisciplinary team must be available for support, counseling, and advice. This team may include doctor, nurse, social worker, clergyman, and lawyer.

---

* For the formulation of this list I am indebted to Dr. Cicely Saunders and Dr. Sylvia Lack.

- The patient should be treated as a person, not as a disease, by professional health-care givers, family, and friends.
- Humanistic care should be integrated with expert medical and nursing care.
- A family facing the impending death of a loved member needs support and advice from health-care professionals.
- The terminal patient must be allowed to give as well as receive.
- We must perpetuate among the dying their continuing self-respect and identity as persons with freedom from being a burden to others.
- The family must feel a sense of participation in care giving and decisionmaking.
- The primary care person tending to a patient at home needs support and occasional relief from duties to the dying person.

The hospice program has evolved in part as an attempt to compensate for the inadequacies of the present medical system, acute-care hospitals, and physicians in relieving the physical distress of the terminal cancer patient. At present, there is but a slim prospect that the average terminal patient suffering from pain in our society will find complete relief. Analgesic dosages (medications that produce insensibility to pain) are generally standardized and seldom graded to meet the patient's individual needs. Anxiety is provoked by anticipation of the cyclic return of pain, the inevitable consequence of inappropriate administration of drugs. Scheduling and apportioning of pain-relieving medications are seldom suited to the patient's requirements; the patient is often sentenced to pass through consecutive stages of sedation, uneasiness, and intense suffering. Narcotics prescribed to be given when needed are often withheld by members of the medical staff to avoid addiction; they are seldom administered before the patient is in a state of acute distress. The result can be inadequate relief of pain, and decreasing potential for the goals of pain control.[7]

Not all cancer patients experience pain, but it is a predominant characteristic of the disease. Hospice is especially helpful to those in a terminal phase of cancer, for the disease is characterized by a lengthy terminal phase and highly distressing symptoms, which may range from difficulty in breathing to difficulty in eating or elimination. Treatment itself produces discomfort, such as the nausea and vomiting associated with chemotherapy. Hospice helps all who suffer from a prolonged terminal illness, but cancer patients are the most common and make up 94 percent of those hospice serves.

That the terminal cancer patient's physical distress is not adequately controlled in the acute care of a general hospital was documented by Dr. Richard Lamerton,[8] who discovered in his study of terminal care that one-fifth of all hospitalized terminal cancer patients are in severe pain. Accounts of the accomplishments of the staff at St. Christopher's Hospice in London contrast markedly with the stated results of other efforts at pain control. In a study of fifteen hundred patients admitted to St. Christopher's for treatment, Dr. Lamerton found that 99 percent of patients with severe pain at the time of their admission were afforded relief following their entry into the service program. Dr. Lamerton affirms as well that the pain experienced by those being cared for at home could be markedly reduced by introducing a hospice home care team and outpatient clinic into the patient's total care regimen. He shows that the terminal patient is more efficiently and properly cared for under hospice guidance than in the general hospital or by the family practitioner at home.[9] This is due at least in part to the willingness of hospice staff to deal with the emotional needs that influence a patient's perception of pain.

Dr. Cicely Saunders maintains that, in addition to the pain caused directly by the malignancy, cancer patients are subject to pain from symptoms that are by-products of the disease or its treatment. Moreover, the patient's perception and experience of pain are strongly influenced by his emotional responses.[10] Relief of pain in the terminally ill is thus a multifaceted problem which requires attendance to the physical pain, the perception of the sensation, and the patient's emotional reaction to it. Dr. Saunders finds that an expression of interest in each patient's particular problems may eliminate much of the physical distress. The presence of a caring figure who listens and attempts to understand the sensation of pain the patient is experiencing is perhaps one of the most important factors in the relief of that pain.

Other noted physicians, such as Dr. Elisabeth Kübler-Ross, have also found that the vigilant presence of someone who is willing to spend time visiting and listening to the patient is a fundamental need of the terminally ill. But since health-care professionals find death extremely threatening, they seek to avoid their dying patients,[11] often relegating them to back rooms, where they are left alone and ignored for extended periods of time. There is a general tendency for members of the medical and nursing staff to avoid eye contact with patients and limit interaction to brief, task-oriented episodes. Physicians make perfunctory and hasty rounds, frequently in groups of two or three, thereby intimidating the patient and eliminating opportunities for communication.[12] When the patient suffering a malignancy is found to be incurable, the physician commonly requests that the chaplain make regular visits and subsequently withdraws his own presence.[13] Because of such general avoidance of dying patients by the health-care staff, treatment of the emotional dimensions of pain is usually neglected. The consequences of such neglect are further compounded by the special problems of chronic pain.

Experience with acute pain cannot be extrapolated to derive an understanding of chronic pain, which is perpetual and progressive rather than transient and reversible. The mental attitude is likely to be quite different, for with acute pain, which is likely to be temporary, a person can summon the strength for endurance while looking forward to the future. A person suffering with chronic pain, which is likely to get worse, may summon the needed strength to endure but may also feel a kind of hopeless resignation, or anger. His whole consciousness may be dominated by pain, which colors everything else in the patient's world.

Physical, psychological, interpersonal, financial, and spiritual factors are among the components of chronic pain, and the complex interaction of these factors creates a situation which Dr. Saunders has termed "total pain." Such pain appears to be needless, and since it occurs as an adjunct to advanced malignant disease, it often forcibly reminds the patient of his terminal prognosis, thereby intensifying his distress. Anticipation of extended episodes of pain leads to anxiety, depression, and insomnia for the terminal patient, and these in turn aggravate the physical component of the pain. In addition, other physical problems, such as bedsores, constipation, cystitis, and musculoskeletal difficulties, tend to occur, though not as a consequence of the malignant process, and demand specific treatment. Effective relief of a terminal patient's discomfort is therefore a multidimensional task which calls for the collaborative effort of an interdisciplinary team in controlling pain and delivering proper nursing care.

Actually ascertaining the individual's particular nursing needs is the first step in attempting to alleviate his pain. The hospice team should take the time to train a "primary care" person—a member of the patient's family, or a friend—to perform these tasks. The primary care person tends to the patient's needs at home, gives medication, and does whatever the home-care situation requires. Educating the patient, the primary care person, and the family in the aspects of nursing care the patient will require is of basic importance in providing optimal comfort. Frequent positional changes are required for the bedridden, to eliminate the possibility of bedsores; proper dietary habits must be introduced to prevent constipation or gastrointestinal distress; a limited amount of exercise should be advised for the nonambulatory to prevent the onset of musculoskeletal pain, and for the ambulatory to ensure that they maintain maximum mobility. Many of the discomforts that present themselves as common symptoms of malignant disease can be mitigated by combining the cooperative skills of nurses and concerned family members. Anorexia, which taxes the patient's general stamina and morale, may be alleviated with appetite increasers, such as glucocortico-steroids, and attention to the patient's dietary preferences. Intractable vomiting or nausea, whether due to a potent narcotic painkiller, a tumorous obstruction, bleeding from a cancerous growth, biochemical upset, or pressure on the gastrointestinal tract, may be meliorated with antiemetics. Difficulty in swallowing may be relieved with local anesthetics and careful attention and assistance while the patient is drinking cool fluids. Dehydration, hiccups, itching, insomnia, urinary complications, and fungating growths similarly should not plague the dying patient if prompt and effective relief can be provided.

When pain cannot be alleviated through nursing techniques alone, and when diversional activity such as occupational therapy, physical therapy, entertainment, and mild forms of recreation prove to be of no avail, the use of analgesic agents may be called for in providing relief to the terminal patient. Non-narcotic analgesics such as aspirin and Tylenol may be quite effective, and are the substances most likely to be prescribed initially for pain relief. If the non-narcotics prove insufficient in controlling the patient's pain, a synthetic narcotic analgesic is often substituted, such as methadone, which is a chemical substitute for plant-derived morphine. Nausea and vomiting, especially with patients in the advanced stages of cancer, are commonly associated with the use of narcotics. To counteract such discomforting side effects, an antiemetic is often prescribed concurrently.

If the patient's pain becomes so severe that the synthetic narcotics fail to provide sufficient analgesia, morphine (in the United States) or diamorphine (in the United Kingdom) may be prescribed by the hospice physician. Caution is urged in the use of narcotic analgesics, and many physicians and medical sources have issued warnings about the danger of tolerance, addiction, and diminishing awareness in the patient.

To determine whether narcotic analgesia led to the impairment of mental faculties or the development of tolerance or addiction, Dr. R. G. Twycross reviewed five hundred patients admitted consecutively to St. Christopher's Hospice in London with advanced malignant disease. From his observation of these patients, he concluded that drowsiness and detachment from reality are related more to advanced physical disability than to administration of a particular narcotic dosage.[14] Twycross also stated that the necessity for increase in narcotic dose is caused more by increased pain than by tolerance; the majority of upward adjustments in diamorphine dosage were for pain associated with different cancerous spreading (metastatic) lesions. Even the development of physical dependence prevents neither a gradual downward adjustment of dose nor the cessation of treatment if the clinical situation warrants it. However, with oral administration of morphine, as in the Brompton narcotic mixture prescribed by hospice physicians, dependence develops less rapidly and possibly to a lesser degree.

Nonetheless, the majority of physicians who care for the terminally ill harbor fears of addiction, tolerance, and mental impairment in their patients, and consequently prescribe narcotics on a four-hourly PRN basis. As I have described, under this system of narcotic administration the patient must be in pain before he is able to receive the drug; if his therapeutic regimen calls for painkiller every four hours and he demonstrates a need for pain-relieving medication before that time has elapsed, he is left to suffer out the remaining interval in pain. The practice at St. Christopher's, and at American hospices, in contrast, is to adjust the level of analgesia to the degree of pain experienced by the patient—that is, increase the dosage gradually until the pain is alleviated. The subsequent dose is given before the effects of the previous dose have subsided, thus keeping pain in abeyance.

According to B. M. Mount, director of the Palliative Care Unit at the Royal Victoria Hospital in Montreal, there are several aims in treating the intractable pain of advanced cancer.[15] Clarification of the cause of the pain is an essential first aim in symptom control and may suggest possible modes of therapeutic intervention. Awareness of the cause of the pain and of the existence of effective therapies for its relief serves to remove the patient from the characteristic state, described by LeShan, of meaninglessness, helplessness, and hopelessness.[16] A second important aim is the anticipation and prevention of pain, as opposed to treatment of pain once it has occurred.

A third aim in the treatment of pain is achieving a pain-free state without sedation. Many patients feel that the only alternatives open to them are constant pain on the one hand and perceptual drowsiness on the other. Comfort and an unclouded mind can be achieved simultaneously, however, if careful individual regulation of analgesic dosage is provided. The ability to relate to his environment in a normal manner, without being groggy from drugs or distressed by inadequate painkiller, is vital to the patient's need. Even the mode of administration should be considered with the maximum benefit to the patient in mind; for example, oral analgesia provides a degree of mobility and independence that is not afforded by IVs.

There is convincing evidence that the Brompton narcotic mixture—a well-known British oral narcotic preparation of diamorphine, cocaine, gin, sugar syrup, and chlorpromazine syrup—is an effective method for the control of severe pain. The mixture is used when milder narcotic and non-narcotic preparations prove ineffective; yet in spite of its potent analgesic effects, it is still useful when a longer survival period is anticipated.[17] With careful monitoring of the patient's needs and adjustment of dosage, the mixture may be used for many months and even several years without dose escalation. In a study of the effects of the Brompton mixture at McGill University in Montreal, the cheerful and friendly environment of a palliative-care unit apparently harmonized with the painkilling effects of the narcotic medication to provide optimal pain relief.[18] Much of the pain of cancer is not an inevitable consequence of the disease, but can be meliorated if doctors are willing to depart from the traditional medical practices of only medicating at the onset of pain.

The terminal illness of a family member can be a source of physical, social, and emotional stress for the rest of the family. Providing care during the night, with consequent loss of sleep, is frequently cited. Outside help in caring for the patient, either during the day or at night, would remedy such physical strain and help the family to give more attention and energy to the patient in care giving. Hospice support can often make a vital difference, as trained volunteers make home visits and give relief to the primary care person.

It is the twenty-four-hour service availability offered by hospices that enables many families to keep the patient at home. Since emergencies often occur at night and on weekends, when traditional medical help is difficult to obtain, family and patient feel more relaxed and secure if they know that help will be forthcoming when needed. The fear and anxiety caused by crises (especially when help is not available) cause some families to give up home care. A family that has gone through a traumatizing incident without help is not likely to risk another. One woman tried in vain to reach her mother's physician for three days, during which the patient had severe bleeding. After admitting her mother to the emergency room, the daughter could not be persuaded to take her home again. The doctor's assurances failed to overcome the fear and anxiety she'd experienced.[19]

The diverse needs of a dying patient and his family—social, spiritual, and physical—call for the support of a multidisciplinary team. Openness and trust prevail with real teamwork, and regular conferences about the needs of each patient and his family ensure this. Frequent communication also prevents duplication of services and any rivalries. The philosophy of an extended team, with the welfare of the patient as the common goal, includes volunteers and the supply staff, even secretaries. Patients and families come to know all the staff, and every staff member is involved in care. Many families have felt grateful to a kind and conscientious secretary. The team concept, with cooperation and ease of communication, enhances unity and the full use of each member's skills. One does not observe the phenomenon of the reverse hierarchy, where the friendliest and most concerned personnel are at the bottom of the professional ladder, as in many hospitals (where orderlies and students may be the only smiling and talkative staff the patient sees). Every member of the hospice team shows concern and interest in the individual patient.

The high level of personal care found in hospices is due largely to the efforts of trained volunteers. Nearly every hospice in this country has volunteers involved in its program. Hospice, Inc., New Haven, has many volunteer R.N.s and L.P.N.s—licensed practical nurses—but all receive up to ten hours of orientation and fieldwork with hospice nurses before being given individual assignments. Volunteers without a medical background are just as valuable and serve in many capacities. After interviews, careful screening, orientation, and training, volunteers are given assignments based on their talents and preferences. Volunteers may serve as direct care givers, receptionists, public speakers, photographers and writers, researchers, leaders of volunteer teams for specific tasks, hosts and hostesses for special events, etc. Volunteers do not replace paid staff, but do provide needed support and supplement the services hospice is able to offer.

Perhaps one of the most valued functions of a volunteer is as a friend. Family and patient may have an easier time relating to and confiding needs to the volunteer, who is often seen as a peer, than to the professional staff. Volunteers may provide much-needed relief for the primary care person, or afford other members of the family equally needed attention. Whatever the services they provide, all volunteers are treated equally among themselves and the professional staff. "Volunteers are respected here more than at any other agency I know," says Sue Cox, former director of volunteers at Hospice, New Haven, "and this is an important part of our team program. We review our work daily, then meet in a team conference every Tuesday, which includes the social worker, the physicians, and all nursing staff. . . . Other agencies in the area . . . do wonder, I think, at all our *listening* to patients! And this is why we allow a great deal of latitude in the hours and times our people work. . . . It is important for them to have time off, because in the case of the hospice volunteer, the gift is so much greater—it is, in a very real sense, the gift of one's self."[20] Unquestionably, volunteers supply much of the warmth of the hospice.

## Why Do We Need Hospice?

Although it is clichéd today to say that we live in a highly technological, bureaucratic society in which community and personal supports and traditions are broken down, nonetheless it's true. The needs of the dying and their families are personal and those needs are not often met by the impersonal, highly specialized medical technology and the bureaucracy of the modern acute-care hospital.

Care should enable the terminal patient to continue as a maximally functioning participant in life, and to maintain his identity and capacity to contribute as a full human being. Unfortunately, dying patients are often cared for in acute-care hospitals and institutional settings in which the structure, organization, and philosophy of the medical staff are geared toward aggressive, curative intervention. Practices in such facilities characteristically exclude the elements that are essential in the delivery of proper terminal care: involvement of the family in the patient's medical situation, which facilitates acceptance and alleviates potential guilt; care of the patient and his family with respect to all relevant needs—physical, emotional, spiritual, and social; avoidance of heroic measures when such treatments are not warranted by the prognosis; effective use of narcotics for the abolition of pain; execution of the patient's wishes with respect to his environment and therapy; integration of the medical staff as a unified team into the process of maintaining the patient's total well-being.

There is general accord among those examining current practices in the care of the terminally ill that such care is usually deficient, inappropriate, limited, and in many cases devastating to the patient. David Shephard cites three reasons for the pervasive inadequacy of terminal care.[21] First, the emphasis on treatment and investigation leads the practitioner to regard the patient as a disease entity and not as a whole person. As Kübler-Ross has illustrated, the patient "may cry for rest, peace and dignity but he will get infusions, transfusions, a heart machine or tracheotomy, if necessary.[22] The patient is often inappropriately subjected to the rigors of curative therapy even when he is beyond the stage of possible recovery, although therapy at such a point should be geared solely to the maximization of comfort. A second factor in deficient terminal care is treatment in an inappropriate environment. In an acute-care hospital, the orientation of facilities, policies, and staff is toward cure rather than palliation, whereas a hospice is by nature dedicated to meeting the everyday needs of its patients. Inadequate care may also be a consequence of the psychological inability of people in our society to confront the dying. Ironically, investigators have found that physicians are more fearful of death than members of any other occupation. Feifel has postulated that practicing curative medicine facilitates and reinforces the denial of death, thereby preventing physicians from comforting their patients and providing nonclinical, social, and personal support.[23]

The third factor underlying inadequate care in a health-care environment is the training of the staff, which exacerbates rather than alleviates societal inability to confront or cope with death. Dehumanizing approaches to patient care result when staff anxieties intervene in the process of assisting the dying person. Defensive behavior such as indifference, hostility, or detachment from the dying person on the part of staff and friends magnifies the loneliness of hospitalization and accentuates withdrawal of the patient, who is already experiencing a diminished sense of self and decreasing awareness of environment. Interaction between patient and staff are strained further by the pressures of bureaucratic hospital procedures.

The tendency to quietly forget about the patient once he is stigmatized with the label "incurable" can bring on a terrible sense of desolation. The patient may become overwhelmed with hopelessness, withdrawing in loneliness and depression.

Death, in the acute-care setting, represents a technological failure, not a natural and inevitable conclusion to life. Fortunately, due in part to the catalytic effects of Elisabeth Kübler-Ross's work, attitudes toward death are being reexamined, and with new attitudes come a more humane and sensible approach to the care of the dying. To accomplish this completely, changes must be made in medical education. Unfortunately, though many enter medical professions for humanitarian reasons, doctors are often trained to cure and not care. "What's happening in our medical schools and hospitals these days?" asks Dr. Morris Wessel, clinical professor of pediatrics at Yale University School of Medicine and a founding member of the New Haven hospice. "You walk to the door, you leave your humanity outside. . . . Why did physicians stop paying attention to the human side of the patient? . . . We need to stop separating our professional functions into little niches in the hospitals and in the medical schools, in the office or home. . . . The young doctors today need to understand that human beings die. It happens; that's reality."[24] Caring is healing, no matter how long the patient lives.

Hospices have an educational effect upon physicians. When the hospice is housed in an institutional setting, physicians in other areas of the hospital have an opportunity to learn about palliative care, about the value of home visits and of interacting with their dying patients. Physicians who continue to care for their patients after referral to an independent hospice are also learning these techniques. Naturally, other aspects of their practice are affected as well. With the comfort of the patient in mind, not only his cure, physicians and nurses become willing to learn about symptom control from hospice.

As the comfort of the patient is one of the prime reasons for hospice, it is also one of the reasons for its popularity. Besides, many people prefer to die at home rather than in an institution. The patient's comfort does not rely exclusively on medications for pain, or on corrective measures for distressing symptoms; it is also drawn from the environment—comfortable, familiar surroundings, loving care, and perhaps two kinds of visitors seldom seen in an acute-care setting: young children and pets. Comfort may also mean the freedom to live and die in the style of life the patient has created.

The comfort of familiar surroundings, or a homelike inpatient hospice unit, benefits the family also. For the patient in distress is not the only one suffering; the family suffers as well. One of the basic tenets of hospice care is the treatment of patient and family together. Death in acute-care institutions has provoked a coming apart for many families; hospice helps to make death a coming together. Approaching death can be spiritual and growth-filled, an experience families can share. Hospice staff are trained to facilitate communication between family members so that the remaining time can be as complete as possible. Family problems cannot be ignored, for if they remain unresolved they affect the peace of the dying patient. When family members are able to express feelings, patients feel less isolated and freer to express their feelings too.

Caring for the patient at home decreases any feelings of guilt the family may have. Even when a patient is cared for in an inpatient hospice unit, the staff encourages family members to attend the patient. Again, training one or more family members as primary care persons lessens the anxiety and stress of patient and family. The family knows that they have done everything they were capable of for the patient's comfort.

Caring for the patient at home also affords the survivors in the family protection from the hazards of bereavement. A recent study indicates that a significant difference exists in the mortality experience of grieving families, depending upon whether the patient died at home or in the hospital. The risk of the closest relative's dying within a year of bereavement was found to double if the first death occurred in a hospital rather than at home.[25] For those cases in which the patient was cared for at home prior to his death, the ability of family members to resist a devastating and prolonged period of grief is attributable to the continuing support of professionals who assisted in the care of the patient, to lessened difficulty in accepting the reality of the loved one's death by those who witnessed the progression of the illness, and to the value of anticipatory grief.

The terminally ill person who is dying at home is still part of the community, a community of neighbors of varying ages and occupations, from the postman to a visiting toddler. It is beneficial for relatives and children to witness the dying process at home, and not be frightened of it. A positive experience at home can counteract the unnatural scenes of violent death that saturate the media. Anyone who has been present during a peaceful death will fear his own mortality less.

After death has occurred, surviving family members receive continued care from hospice. Hospices in this country and in England offer individual bereavement support, follow-up visits by hospice staff, and bereavement groups. This helps to prevent some of the loneliness which exacerbates grief. Mourners often experi-

ence isolation, and do not receive much understanding or tolerance from the rest of society. After the first flurry of activity
following a death, the bereaved are likely to be left alone, and are
expected to return to "normal" within a short time. We are beginning to recognize, however, along with changing attitudes toward
death, that mourning is a necessary psychological process which
can be aided by acknowledgment from the rest of the community.
Hospices are invaluable in this process, for the family, as the unit
of care, is not abandoned after a member's death. The bereavement process cannot be avoided or curtailed, but it can be resolved
by continuity of care.

We often think of the dying as "them" and the living as "us," as
if we were separate. Among the moral and spiritual benefits of
caring for a dying family member is the erasure of this distinction.
We are all on the same journey, come from the same entrance and
leave by the same exit. We are all wayfarers on the road, and all of
us need to stop for refreshment and comfort before the end of our
journey. With hospice, we now have a choice about where and
how we would like that stop to be.

# 2 ❧
# Types of Hospice Care

## Home-Care Programs

Hospice home-care programs aim to satisfy the psychological, physiological, spiritual, and social needs of the dying. By employing specialized, intensive medical, nursing, and pharmaceutical services, the treatment program is directed at controlling pain, nausea, and other symptoms related to terminal disease which deprive the patient of strength needed to participate in living. Such symptoms management enhances the quality of life by enabling the patient to remain comfortable, alert, and in good spirits during his last days, and eliminating a preoccupation with suffering. The hospice staff, as witnesses to disruption of the family life style by multiple changes which occur during the course of terminal illness, recognize the importance of sustaining continuity of care. Because terminal illness upsets the equilibrium of the family group, it is the patient-family unit which is designated for care. Medical attention and supportive counseling involve both patient and family by day in their homes. The team is also on call for emergencies at night and on weekends. A vital aspect of maintaining family cohesion is the training of a "primary care person" in nursing methods, enabling his or her active participation in and valuable contribution to the care of the patient. In addition, hospice volunteer services free more time for the family to draw closer to the patient and to themselves. By thus incorporating the family into the patient-care system, the anguish of loneliness and isolation experienced by the patient is reduced, and the ability of the hospice team to provide support for the family before, during, and after the patient's death is greatly enhanced.

The specific goals of the hospice home-care program are:

- To aid in reducing the burden of a traumatic life experience by sharing and meeting the expressed needs (physical, emotional, spiritual, and social) of patient and family.
- To assist the patient in achieving and maintaining maximum independent living, with dignity, until death.
- To minimize the painful and damaging effects of the death of a family member upon the family that remains.

Basic to the hospice home-care system is belief in the right of the terminal patient to die at home.

By integrating humanistic, medical, and nursing care, hospice home care attempts to provide a warm atmosphere of peace and friendliness in which the patient can ask questions about his condition. Hospice is concerned with teaching health professionals and relatives that evasion and deception only exacerbate the patient's difficulty in coping with his condition. It is essential that staff and patient alike are prepared to confront the whole truth about the patient's imminent death, and that the staff is ready to listen openly and supportively to the patient as the final stages of his life and illness are resolved.

Maintenance of the family as a cohesive, supportive unit, provision for the relief of loneliness and separation anxiety, and symptom control for the maximum comfort and alertness of the dying patient are key objectives of the hospice staff in assuring accessibility of professional and auxiliary staff skills and in making arrangements for optimum care in a home environment.

If the needs of the family of the patient are inadequately attended to, attempts at meaningful care of the patient may be in vain. Thus, orientation toward both patient and family is a basic tenet of the hospice endeavor, and consideration of the family, often reluctant to disclose its own needs, is accepted as an essential component of home care. Only when feelings of anger, guilt, and loneliness experienced by family members are vented and dissipated can the unspoken sense of alienation in the dying patient be alleviated. Family problems are often too closely related to interaction with the terminally ill patient to go unheeded.

Patients' behavioral patterns frequently undergo a marked change, and overlapping manifestations of denial and depression dominate their relationships with others. At this time the medical team, and more especially the family members, desperately need to understand that a patient's changed behavior is not a result of something they may or may not have done but a predictable response to a very difficult situation.

The hospice home-care team gives the family, and the primary care person in particular, support for the care given the patient. Families may compare themselves with professionals and doubt their capacity to care for the patient even though they desire to do so. Realistic reassurance by a professional can give the family the confidence they need in order to continue. As one woman attested: "Dr. Martinson would constantly reassure us that his care was as good, if not better, than he would receive in the hospital. And how I needed that reassurance—I knew Eric wanted to be at home but I was by no means all that confident that I was enterprising enough to handle it." Dr. Ida Martinson noted later that the primary care person considered her own care inadequate, "though in reality it was excellent."[1]

Families can offer excellent care and can meet the demands of trying situations creatively. Pain is controlled in the home not only be medications administered by the family but also by other means: fantasy, relaxation, diversion, sensory stimulation (massage, patting, and touching). Intravenous feeding is supplanted in the home by frequently offered favorite beverages. Failing appetites are encouraged by familiar foods. The confidence the family members feel in their ability to deliver care is reinforced by the patient's satisfaction in being home, by the comments of professionals, and by the twenty-four-hour backup of the hospice home-care team.

The family also gains confidence through the education and preparation given by the home-care team. Families and patients achieve control over their situation through information on likely side effects of various drugs and knowledge of complications that are likely to arise, as well as preparations to make. Imagined crises are less fearful when patient and family know how to deal with them should they occur. Gathering supplies for possible crises (such as extra towels for hemorrhaging) also helps the family feel more control; whatever is predictable and acted upon lessens fear of the unknown.

Since patient and family are regarded as the unit of care, one of the requirements for acceptance into most hospice home-care programs is the presence of a primary care person in the home, yet this requirement is sometimes handled flexibly. A patient with no relative who can serve as a primary care person may be able to remain at home supported by a network of friends, neighbors, or church groups who can provide twenty-four-hour care. "Family," in these situations, extends to the community, and reminds us of the concept of hospitality in hospice.

Other requirements for admission into a hospice home-care program include a life prognosis of six months or less, understanding on the part of the patient and the family that no resuscitation attempts will be made, a desire for the services hospice provides, and the continued involvement and cooperation of the referring physician (whenever possible).

Home-care staffs provide a variety of services to patients and families. Their visits fall into the following categories:

- Assessment or evaluation
- Physical care
- Teaching
- Social service
- Pastoral
- Death pronouncement
- Bereavement
- Discharge[2]

Home-care staffs need to make many assessment or evaluation visits, as the patient's condition changes continually during a terminal illness. As the disease progresses, there may be almost daily, or at least weekly, changes in the patient's physical and emotional states. Frequent visits are needed to keep the patient comfortable and to help the family through times of rapid change and stress.

Home-care teams in hospices throughout the country offer bereavement follow-up for families as a final service to the patient. Both professionals and trained volunteers make visits after death and on into the mourning period, depending upon the needs of the family. This important work acts as a form of physical and social preventive medicine. Unassisted, grief has vast consequences for the bereaved and for society. Some of the possible aftereffects in the first year following bereavement include: alcoholism, depression, increased vulnerability to illness (there is a 40 percent increase in the mortality rate for widowers), long-term detrimental effects to children caused by the loss of a parent,[3] decreased income and financial difficulties if the head of the household dies, and an increased divorce rate among parents who have lost a child. Some of the common somatic expressions of grief are: sighing, restlessness, insomnia, swallowing, increased or decreased appetite, fatigue. What can be done to alleviate some of the suffering and pain survivors experience after a major loss?

Those trained in hospice care (and many others) recognize that grief is a process, a necessary one, which must be gone through in order to integrate the loss and accommodate any changes in the personality due to this loss. Grief is not an illness which can be drugged and sedated. Mourning is a time of spiritual and emotional need, in which the survivor is adjusting to a markedly altered environment and role change (from wife to widow, from husband to widower, from parents to a family without a child or without a seriously ill child). Dr. Colin Murray Parkes has conducted many studies on bereavement, and found a number of factors, both before and after a death, that aid or hinder the resolution of grief.

The patients' and families' environment before the death influence the survivors' health later. For instance, in a study of widows, those who suffered the greatest emotional disturbance had not been able to prepare themselves for bereavement, had inhibited their own reaction to impending loss in order to "protect" their dying spouse. In these situations the couples grew further and further apart during the illness and each faced the death alone. Dr. Parkes contrasts this situation with couples observed in a hospice-like environment, where it is often possible for a husband and wife to help each other accept approaching death and bereavement.[4] Though these couples did suffer "anticipatory" grief, they were able to achieve a calm period of contentment which persisted until the death and after. Survivors were able later to look back upon this period with satisfaction, and experienced less guilt and remorse than those who had not been able to communicate freely.

An environment in which death is seen as a meaningful event, and in which the psychological and spiritual needs of the patient are the concern of the medical staff, helps to create a setting in which fears and griefs can be discussed. Such a setting is a "safe" place to die. Also, those who have been able to share their thoughts and ideas for the future, who have been able to begin to imagine a life without the dying family member, and who have made practical preparations, are better able to cope with bereavement. When families know that there are others around who will help the survivors, it is easier for them to enjoy their remaining time together.

Dr. Parkes's research has enabled many hospices to determine which family members are likely to be "high risk"—those who may have the greatest difficulty with bereavement. For example, a high risk might be a young widow with several young children at home, who had experienced depression in the past and had been greatly dependent upon her husband. However, a person could have all these factors and yet not experience difficulty, or have none of these factors and encounter difficulties. Yet, the hospice team is able to predict quite accurately whether or not any family members are likely to experience difficulties in bereavement.

The professional hospice team, and regular volunteers, have

usually gotten to know the family well throughout the time of illness, so when death occurs, they are "like family." Some members of the team, often the nurse and volunteers, usually attend the funeral and visit again later. Further visits may be made as called for, depending upon family needs. Dr. Parkes found that widows who had not been permitted to talk about their husband's death, or to express their feelings, suffered a greater loss of health.[5] Families may have unanswered questions haunting their minds, questions that can add to their burdens if not asked and aired. Given the opportunity, the surviving spouse or parent may be eager to ask: "Did we do the right thing? Would he/she have lived if we'd known the diagnosis earlier?" The hospice home-care nurse is a comfortable person to share these concerns with, and can lighten the hearts and minds of the bereaved. A nurse or hospice volunteer who has become "like family" is a sympathetic friend who can give the family needed reassurance and validation of their experience. The emotions of bereavement may be quite a new experience (even if anticipatory grief occurred), and the mourners may need reassurance that their feelings and thoughts are "normal." People meet the needs of their grief in individual ways—by wearing the lost spouse's wedding ring, perhaps, or some item of clothing, by giving away or keeping a loved child's toys—and are helped by "permission" to meet these needs. The family and the hospice team have experienced a peaceful death together, and together they can share the spiritual benefits. Discussing the events of the terminal illness and death diminishes the ill effects of grief and soothes the heart in spite of its sadness. The hospice team will also experience some sadness, for they will have gotten to know and appreciate the dying person. The personal interest and affection the hospice staff demonstrates for the deceased are a comfort to the surviving family. Together they affirm that the deceased's life and individuality had meaning.

The grief process can be a lonely one, and many people find it easier to talk with someone who has gone through the same experience. Well-meaning friends and relatives, important as they are, often are at a loss for words unless they have experienced a similar bereavement. Sometimes family members are too involved in their own grief to be able to help each other. For these reasons, many hospices offer bereavement support groups, which include patients' families as well as a trained counselor. Families help each other, and those whose bereavement is more distant can share valuable insight and practical advice with the newly bereaved. There is a link of understanding through a shared experience among the bereaved which transcends other differences. Self-help bereavement groups are also an opportunity for members to give to each other, and to share the spiritual gifts gathered during a peaceful death. Many of the contacts between families begin prior to the bereavement support group, among those who have met informally at the inpatient hospice unit.

One family I worked with in Connecticut chose the hospice home-care program because they liked the accessibility of doctors and nurses on the staff and wanted to be able to talk about their needs freely. They were an old New England family, and greatly preferred the privacy of their home to a hospital. Even at home they desired privacy and wished to do things in their own way, without interference. For these reasons, they liked the flexibility of a hospice nurse, who would be there only when needed.

Mrs. Butterworth was fifty-four, and dying of cancer of the breast which had spread extensively throughout her body. Calm and unemotional about death, she generally behaved like a "brave soldier." She openly discussed death with acceptance and used her remaining time to "put her house in order." Her concern about drug addiction necessitated reassurance about the medications she used. She was also concerned about her husband, who had begun drinking during her illness, and was reassured that the hospice bereavement team would look after him.

Mr. Butterworth was a reserved, stoical Yankee, and hard to talk to. He rarely mentioned his own feelings, but would reply if questioned by members of the hospice team. He was very supportive of his wife's care at home, but generally did not participate. Mrs. Butterworth was cared for by her sister. Though Mr. Butterworth did not perform direct care himself, he visited and spent time with his wife and never neglected to bring her fresh flowers every day.

The couple had several grown children with families of their own. They were not involved in their mother's direct care, but visited her and talked with the hospice social worker.

Mrs. Butterworth died peacefully at home, as she had wished, in the company of her sister and her husband. She concluded her life well, leaving no unfinished business. Her husband received follow-up care from the bereavement team, particularly visits from volunteers. His drinking did not increase, and as his wife had predicted, he began dating less than a year after her death. The family (sister, grown children, and husband) were all satisfied with the hospice home-care program and were glad they had been able to talk freely with their beloved sister, mother, and wife.

Another family consulted several times with me and other members of the staff of Hospice, Inc., New Haven, then finally decided upon an acute-care hospital. Mr. Ziccarelli was an Italian in his sixties, dying of cancer, but the choice was made by his wife and three voluble daughters. They decided against hospice, for to them hospice care meant giving up, meant the end, meant death. The mother and the daughters were fearful of death and wanted the patient to continue aggressive therapy. The family warned us not to use the words "cancer" and "hospice" in front of the patient, and tried to convince themselves that he was not dying (though the cancer had spread throughout his body and he was in the terminal phase of the disease).

Also, the family did not want him home and did not want to be involved in his care themselves. Later, when he was hospitalized, family members avoided going to visit as he grew closer to death. The family also chose the hospital because of the technology available there, for they were still hoping for a cure and looking for a miracle to save him.

Mother and daughters maintained denial until his death. Follow-up was done by the hospital social worker, who noted that the family had great difficulties after bereavement. Fighting split the family apart and all felt guilty over unresolved issues.

Not all families grow together during a terminal illness, and not all patients find acceptance, as Mrs. Butterworth did. Hospice care, and home-care programs, are not appropriate for everyone. Cost was not a factor for either of these families. Hospice services are much less expensive than hospitalization, but both families were willing to spend whatever was necessary for what they considered the best possible care.

## Inpatient Hospice Programs

Most hospices in the United States provide a home-care program and bereavement services, but not all have inpatient services, though this is one of the goals of the hospice concept. Inpatient facilities offer a number of advantages for the terminally ill and are free of the restrictions of an acute-care hospital (e.g., visiting restrictions, aggressive therapy, impersonal care, and institutional environment). Inpatient units especially aid:

- Patients who, with additional support, can remain at home.
- People who are unable to cope any longer in their own homes.
- Patients whose symptoms can be alleviated by round-the-clock attention.
- Those whose families, wearied by prolonged nursing, need a rest themselves.
- Those whose families have been unable to take a vacation because of their nursing commitment.

Eligibility requirements are the same for an inpatient and a home-care hospice patient; once admitted to one program, the patient is eligible for the other. In fact, a patient may at times move between the programs, according to his needs. The basic question is always: "What does the patient need, and how can we best meet those needs?" Like the home-care patient, the person admitted to an inpatient facility must have a limited life prognosis, usually of less than six months, and the continued participation of the personal physician who directs the patient's medical management. Hospice physicians serve as consultants to the personal physician in the areas of symptom control and medical management.

Dan is a good example of a patient who utilized both home and inpatient hospice services. He was a young French Canadian, thirty-four years old, with cancer of the colon which had spread extensively. He wanted hospice care more than anything, and very much preferred to die at home. Though his young wife was not as keen on home care as he was, she went along with his decision. She took very good care of him and was loving and supportive.

Not all of Dan's symptoms could be controlled at home, however. He was admitted to the inpatient hospice program in great distress and spent two weeks there. He wanted desperately to go home, and when his symptoms were under control he did. Four days later he died with his wife lying next to him, cradling him in her arms. He died as he had wished, in familiar surroundings. His death was peaceful, unmarred by unresolved issues with his wife or loving thoughts unexpressed.

The couple had a young daughter, who was cared for by her grandmother during Dan's illness. The child was sheltered from the situation, but did have opportunities to visit her father and to say goodbye.

Cost was not a major factor in Dan's decision, for he wanted to die at home, but for this young couple hospice care was the least expensive alternative. The hospice inpatient unit was of critical importance in allowing him to have his death as he wished.

Inpatient hospice facilities appear to be developing in two directions, some independently and some housed in acute-care hospitals. The survey I made with Dale Lupu of a sample of American hospices revealed that of the ten hospices that offered inpatient programs, only two were independent.[6]

Both independent and hospital-based facilities make every effort to provide a home-like atmosphere for the comfort and privacy of patients and families. Independent hospices have more freedom, of course, to design buildings that enhance the hospice concept, and to include features such as small lounges for private conversation, bedrooms for visiting families, kitchens for family use, playgrounds for children, and gardens or private patios for patient and staff enjoyment. While maintaining strict standards of cleanliness, the independent hospice can foster a noninstitutional atmosphere through homelike touches such as hanging plants, wall decorations, and comfortable furniture. Patients are encouraged to bring possessions that have meaning for them. While some medical equipment is kept for patient comfort—oxygen, for example—one will not see imposing-looking medical apparatus or resuscitation equipment. Chapels are usually available for services as well as for the private use of patients and families. Many hospices have a viewing room in which the family can spend some time alone with the deceased.

Hospice units within a hospital setting also decorate in a homelike manner, with cheerful colors and space for families to eat together, and sometimes even to spend the night if they wish. The spirit of the hospice environment is created as much, if not more, by the staff as by the furnishings. Just as important to the patient as light, greenery, and cheerful colors is an atmosphere of acceptance of terminal illness and death, and the unhurried interest of the staff. Patients are known and greeted by name and are not referred to impersonally.

Creating within the hospital setting a hospice environment of care rather than cure, of humane and practical symptom control, takes real determination and dedication on the part of the medical director and staff. Hospital administrators need to understand hospice priorities and philosophy and perceive a need for improvement in the care of the terminally ill, and be willing to make a commitment to the hospice program. The hospice medical director with the hospital needs the administrators' understanding and the freedom to organize services somewhat differently from the rest of the hospital. The medical director also needs to train staff in hospice methods and philosophy and select nurses and aides who are interested in working with the terminally ill and their families.

To accomplish this, Dr. Norman Walter, director of the Kaiser-Permanente Hayward Hospice Pilot Project in Los Angeles, educated physicians to recognize when attention to the comfort of the patient is more appropriate than plans for cure, and to recognize when a patient is within three to six months of death. Physicians, who were used to consulting only other physicians or medical professionals, also learned to be part of a team that includes professionals, volunteers, and the family. They were enabled to discuss impending death with patients and their families. Skills for symptom control and management were upgraded and physicians acquired an understanding and appreciation of the hospice program. Other staff members and volunteers were also instructed in hospice concepts and in their practical application. All were trained to become a team. Every member of the medical center, including administrators, gardeners, housekeepers, and dieticians, was trained and given an orientation to hospice goals and philosophy. This educational program was necessary to change attitudes from fear to acceptance of dying and death. Dr. Walter helped his staff to see that giving such care to the dying could be a satisfying and fulfilling experience.

Another good example of a hospital-based hospice unit is the Palliative Care Unit of the Royal Victoria Hospital in Montreal. This cheerful, friendly unit is staffed by leaders trained at St. Christopher's who give careful attention to pain and symptom control. The staff work well together as a team, and they and the volunteers are dedicated to helping patients and families to live as fully as possible during their remaining time together.

I visited both the surgical ward and the Palliative Care Unit in the role of a patient and found significant differences between the two. So that I would be treated as a patient, and as fully as possible experience the life of a patient, I became one by losing weight, undergoing radiation treatment and biopsy, as well as having my veins punctured to simulate chemotherapy. Having cared for many cancer patients, I had no difficulty in identifying with them or being accepted as one of them. During my ten-day stay at the hospital I began to suffer many symptoms common among cancer patients, including fatigue, appetite loss, and pain. While in the surgical ward, I also experienced a loss of personal identity, common in institutions, as I was referred to by my disease instead of by name. Like other patients, I felt bored and isolated.

Nurses in the Palliative Care Unit (PCU) made more than four times as many visits to talk with me while I was a patient, and each visit was of longer duration and of a much friendlier nature than I experienced on the surgical ward. During the initial nursing interview, I was asked such questions as: "What do you like to eat?" and "Is there anything special you like to do?" The nurse who conducted the interview sat down while we talked so that we could have eye contact. PCU also greeted me, as they do other patients, with a personal note of welcome and flowers by my bedside.

Staff members were as capable and professional as those on the surgical ward, but seemed freer to express their own personalities. On the ward, the smiles were rare and the personalities hidden. Direct orders to patients were common on the surgical ward ("Go back to bed"), but never occurred in the PCU. The attitude of caring, the smiles and personal interest of the staff, created a cheerful atmosphere which the patients commented on.

I also noted that families spent far more time at the bedside of the patient, participating in direct personal care. Staff encouraged the families to visit, and they felt at ease washing and feeding the patient, changing bed linen, bringing a urinal, and smoothing sheets and pillows. On the surgical ward, families were made to feel in the way and spent more time in the visitors' lounge, where they were more at ease. In the PCU, the staff helped families experience death as a deeply meaningful shared event which drew them closer together. Families also found satisfaction by doing kindnesses for the dying members of other families, and through talking and sharing with each other.

In hospices, families tend to comfort each other through each stage of illness and bereavement, for they share similar emotions and experiences. Patients are often able to comfort one another too, for as social masks slip away during illness, friendships can form more quickly on a deeper level. Lack of time is compensated by intensity. "Time," as Dr. Cicely Saunders once said, "is not a question of length, it's a question of depth, isn't it?"

Good hospice care affords the opportunity to reach this depth of experience and to overcome the fear of death. As patients and families witness the peaceful transitions around them, death is seen as part of each soul's journey. In spite of the sadness they feel at parting, these patients and families do not experience death as either terrible or frightening, but as part of the cycle of life.

Peaceful deaths and good care are possible whether the patient is cared for at home with hospice support, in a hospital-based hospice inpatient unit, or in an independent hospice inpatient unit. Services do not differ; however, both independent and exclusively home-care programs tend to offer a greater variety of professional, nonprofessional, and volunteer skills. Together with their wider range of social and psychological services, they have greater freedom and flexibility. Independent hospices have more control over their physical and psychological environment; this is usually reflected in more spacious accommodations and in the "psychological space" needed to create a hospice community.

Both hospital and hospice offer a medical service requiring trained technical skills, but a hospital does not become a hospice just by setting aside a ward for dying patients. Hospices and hospitals have different goals and philosophies of care, and the hospital-based hospice unit must maintain itself as a community amid the impersonal, machine-oriented medical care that surrounds it. The success of the institutionally based hospice (and of the hospice movement in general) is due to the attitudes toward the dying, the concern, dedication, and commitment, of the individuals who have organized and who staff each hospice. Perhaps it is easier to maintain this commitment in an independent, and more reinforcing, environment. With increased awareness, perhaps one day the humanistic rather than the technological attitude toward the patient will come to pervade the hospital.

## Volunteers

Volunteers are an integral part of the hospice team, and are carefully trained and screened before their placement in the most appropriate situation. Listening and communications skills are practiced, and each volunteer becomes familiar with the literature on death and dying as well as the humanistic philosophies that are fundamental to hospice. To hospice the volunteer brings a fresh attitude and outlook, and a renewing perspective from a nonmedical background. It is not necessary to be a professional in order to be a friend to a dying patient, nor is it necessary to be a professional to listen sympathetically to a person in grief. Dying is a social issue which involves the whole human community, and the volunteer, as a member of that community, is well suited to reinforce the support the family and the patient need. Dying patients and their families do not always need counselors or professionals to talk to. As Sylvia Lack, medical director of Hospice, Inc., New Haven, has said: "I don't consider dying a psychiatric disease." A good volunteer becomes a friend of the family and is seen as one of themselves, a peer. Sometimes it is easier for the patient/family to confide in or open up to a volunteer than to a professional. And when a relationship has been developed during illness, the volunteer can become an important visitor during bereavement.

Volunteers add to the richness and variety of hospice programming. They are also important educators in their community, for their own experiences will diminish others' fear of the mystery of death. Hospices become available in communities that want and need them, and work to establish them. Volunteers from the community help to provide the energy and support the hospice needs to exist.

Volunteers also take the burden off the professional staff, and replenish their enthusiasm, preventing staff "burnout." A volunteer who comes in once or twice a week brings a new outlook and can help relieve the stress the staff may feel. After a harried day filled with crises, a nurse may turn to a volunteer for a fresh viewpoint and mental relaxation. In turn, the clinical staff is available to the volunteer to discuss questions or problems. These mutual supports between patient/family, professional, and volunteer make hospice a community. One of the most important factors in hospice care is the people, and volunteers are important people in that care.

## Nursing Homes

St. Christopher's Hospice in London has a section called The Draper's Wing, for elderly residents. It is not a nursing home as we know it in this country (though some of the residents do eventually move to the terminal-care sections of the hospice), but is another example of the St. Christopher's concept of community. The elderly residents are as much a part of this house of life as the children in the play school in St. Christopher's gardens. The hospice is a place of welcome for people of all ages and in all stages on the journey of life.

Nursing homes in the United States are extended-care facilities, usually for the elderly. The usual nursing home here is not likely to have a children's play school and terminally ill patients within the same facility. Though many people do die in extended-care facilities, when they begin to fail they are more likely to be transported to an acute-care hospital to die. Nursing homes provide programs that are ideally suited for the long-term geriatric patient, but are not usually able to cope with the multitude of rapidly changing problems of the dying patient; nor are they willing to deal with the acute crisis of the death itself. Many nursing homes return the patient to the hospital, which results in an unnecessary, expensive journey and high-cost hospital care for the last day or two of life.

Nursing homes provide care for long-term chronic illness which may or may not lead to terminal illness. Care is usually given by untrained nursing assistants supervised by an R.N. with direction from the patient's physician. Nursing assistants may not receive orientation prior to their work with patients and are not usually trained to care for the dying or their families. Much excellent care is given in nursing homes due to the care and concern of the staff, but many of these staff members are paid a minimum wage and have had little training.

In the inpatient hospice, the patient is a member of the hospice team, and he/she can maintain an individual life style. While nursing homes are less rigid about routine than most hospitals, patients must conform to the institutional structure. Days are scheduled, and activities such as meals and baths follow a routine. It is sometimes difficult for new patients to adapt to the patterns of living in the nursing home. Hospice care usually adapts to the patient's pattern of living, with the patient maintaining as much control as possible.

More and more nursing homes make an effort to include the family and recognize the patient's need for family members and for contact with the community. However, this is still a long way from the bringing-together process of hospice patient/family care. Nursing home staff may not be trained to facilitate communication between the patient and the family, or to deal effectively with the needs of family members, particularly during a terminal illness. Families are less likely to participate in the nursing home patient's direct care or to receive bereavement follow-up after the patient's death.

Volunteers add important social contacts to the life of the nursing home patient, but the role is quite different from that of a hospice volunteer. While the volunteer in the nursing home may fill some of the patient's social needs and may act as an advocate for the patient with doctors and nursing staff, he/she seldom gives the patient direct care. The nursing home volunteer is important to the patient, but is not a member of the care team, and is not on a par with the professional staff as is his/her hospice counterpart. Also, like nursing home staff, nursing home volunteers do not receive the training and orientation the hospice volunteer receives, and are not trained to offer support for the patient's family.

While nursing home care may be very good, it still does not provide real hospice care, and it follows different principles. "Nursing home" and "hospice" are not interchangeable; those who use the word "hospice" must provide hospice services.

Hospice philosophy is not confined to any particular institution, however, and a flexible nursing home can adapt many hospice techniques, as was done in the case of Sol. Sol was a Jewish man of eighty-two and had lived happily in the same Bronx nursing home for a number of years. Sol's son consulted me because his father was dying of cancer of the colon, with extensive spreading. Cancer spreads more slowly in the elderly and Sol had had it for several years. Sol's son wanted to be sure his father was receiving the best care possible.

Though Sol was eligible for hospice care, he was happy in the nursing home and wanted to remain. Over the years he had made many friends there and he enjoyed their company. The son's work took him out of town quite frequently and he could not care for his father full-time by himself. There were no other relatives available to care for Sol at home.

The nursing home was also concerned about caring for Sol and was quite willing to learn of any hospice methods that could help him. Hospice nurses visited and educated the nurses; I helped the staff to be aware of Sol's other needs and cautioned them about the feelings of abandonment and isolation the dying often face in institutions. Sol had worked outdoors all his life and his special love was the rose garden. The nursing home was very understanding of his need to garden and made sure that there was an orderly to take him outdoors every day. Sol was able to work in the rose garden daily until five days before his death.

His son was pleased to know that the nursing home staff had been trained by the hospice. The nursing home adapted another hospice ideal, direct care of the patient by the family, for Sol's son spent the last week by his father's bedside. Sol died peacefully, attended by his son to the last.

## Visiting Nurse Associations

Visiting nurse associations, or R.N. services, or home health services—the names for this service vary—are provided through local public health departments and service details may vary from community to community. Visiting nurses provide intermittent care for bedbound patients and also educate the family to provide skin care, give pain medications, etc. Their services are ideal for the home-care patient/family, except that they are usually provided only during working hours, Monday through Friday. Local hospices make an effort not to duplicate services and to work in conjunction with visiting nurses. The hospice can utilize the skills and services of the visiting nurses and vice versa. The care of the terminally ill is a community concern, just as dying is a social issue, and the patient benefits from cooperation between agencies.

In Tucson, Arizona, for example, Home Health Services make referrals to St. Mary's Hospice and ask for consultations on symptom and pain control for some of their cancer patients. The two agencies work together in harmony for the benefit of the terminally ill. The hospice in turn uses the public health physical therapist. Both are hosts and guests, offering and receiving hospitality along with services, which is the core of hospice care.

# 3 ❧
# Hospice Issues and Problems, Development and Administration

I want to discuss here in greater depth and detail the issues and problems raised in earlier chapters, both for the benefit of readers in the health-care field and for lay readers, so that both may understand and evaluate the issues confronting hospice and administrative functioning. Since the health-care professional and the lay person work together as a team in hospice, any issue or problem that affects one affects the other. Both are concerned with translating the ideals of hospice into practical action and each will find the discussions in this chapter useful.

Among staffing issues are administration, the multidisciplinary team, hospice nurses (who might more appropriately be L.P.N.s than R.N.s), staff stress, patient and staff perceptions of "good care," and the director of volunteers. I will go into symptom control as well as the patient's nonphysical needs, such as creativity, socialization, emotional and spiritual sustenance.

In this chapter I will also discuss the necessary issue of reimbursement, the economic considerations furthering institutionally based hospices, and their possible disadvantages. Institutionally based hospices will be compared with independent inpatient hospices and home-care programs. Just as the hospice patient is more than his/her body, so hospice is more than a building, and it is sometimes helpful to examine hospice concepts of care and home-care programs apart from the buildings that facilitate them. There is a need for evaluation of existing hospice programs and for criteria that developing hospices can use for guidelines. I will also describe some of the instances where hospital care is preferred.

Hospice's relationship to the community can further public education about the terminally ill as well as uncover the often suppressed issue of death. Death must not be a hidden issue, and exposure to peaceful deaths, as well as exposure to hospice, can increase public acceptance of its naturalness. Death, for the patients, families, visitors, and staff at hospice, is often very sad, but not terrifying.

Hospice planners should make an effort to work cooperatively with other human-service agencies and health-care programs. Efforts should be made not to duplicate services. Medical fragmentation is expensive and confusing for the patient, and hospice must not further fragment medical care. Hospice integrates many services within its program.

There is a need for regulation to ensure high standards of care and to guarantee that those who use the name "hospice" actually deliver hospice care.

Finally, the welcome popularity of the hospice concept holds some dangers. Perhaps, though, the success of hospice will alter and shape medical care in other settings. Will hospice care become the standard in the future? I certainly hope so.

## The Multidisciplinary Team

Everyone who participates in the patient's care is part of the multidisciplinary team: physician, nurses, social worker, physical therapist, pharmacologist, chaplain, volunteers, patient, and family. Roles within the team vary according to skills, length of employment, education, and title, and are flexibly changing as each staff member grows in experience and skill. Teams function differently around individual patients, for each patient has different needs and will choose to relate to each staff member accordingly. Hospice care is personal and the personal needs and preferences of each patient/family will shape the team. The coordinator of the team is usually the medical director, but it may be the director of nurses.

## Administration

The administration is an important part of the effectiveness of the multidisciplinary team, with the administrator serving as a liaison with the board of directors, the medical director, and the director of the home-care program. The administrator represents the hospice when working with other health-care agencies and when speaking to members of the community. The administrator understands and has a commitment to hospice care and its patients and families. Combining the fundamental caring attitudes of hospice with necessary practicalities, the administrator needs to have skills in public relations and developing funding resources.

## Medical Director

The medical director is a liaison between the hospice and the medical community. The personal physician continues to plan his patient's medical care, but he may consult the medical director regarding symptom control. The medical director may refer the patient to other facilities when appropriate (such as radiation therapy for pain control, or an acute-care setting if needed). The medical director is coordinator of the multidisciplinary team and must have a thorough understanding of the needs of the terminally ill. He/she has a commitment to hospice philosophies of care, and shares this with other members of the team.

Everyone on the staff—physicians, nurses, and other medical personnel—receives training, as I discussed in the previous chapter. All staff members are given help in exploring their own feelings about death and loss, as well as feelings about working with the terminally ill and about palliative care rather than cure.

All of the team (including patients and families) need to understand and accept the concept of palliative care as the major medi-

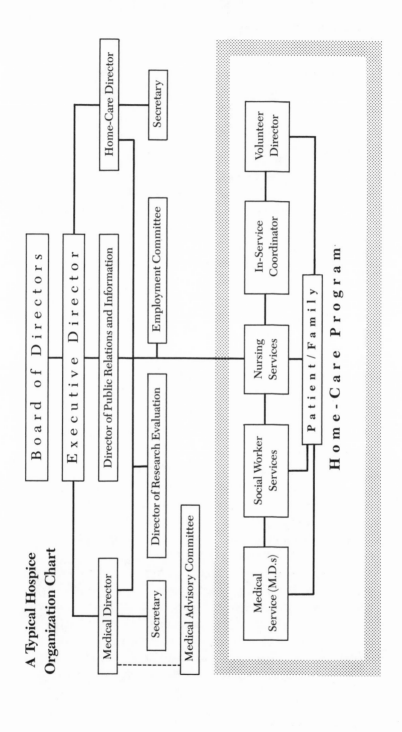

A Typical Hospice
Organization Chart

Board of Directors

Executive Director

Home-Care Director

Secretary

Director of Public Relations and Information

Employment Committee

Director of Research Evaluation

Medical Director

Secretary

Medical Advisory Committee

Home-Care Program

Volunteer Director

In-Service Coordinator

Nursing Services

Social Worker Services

Medical Service (M.D.s)

Patient/Family

cal goal. The inappropriateness of resuscitation attempts and life-prolonging techniques, the acceptance of death—these are fundamental to the basic philosophy of everyone on the team.

## Symptom Control

The team learns to do what is necessary for the patient's comfort. Symptom control is not just for pain; it includes many other things. Good skin care can prevent or clear up bedsores through the use of water mattresses, sheepskin pads, rubs, and frequent changes of position. Good mouth care prevents sores and infections. Bowel function is also important to the bedbound patient. Constipation, a frequent side effect of many analgesics, may be helped by prescriptions (included with the pain medications), enemas, and removal of fecal impaction. There are many distressing symptoms the team needs to be aware of and know how to treat: urinary problems, nausea and vomiting, shortness of breath, coughing, sleep difficulty, diarrhea, edema, ascites (fluid collecting in the abdominal cavity), and itching, to name a few. When cure is no longer possible, there is still much a physician can do. The medical team is skilled in symptom control, and as the whole hospice team learns, the application of hospice philosophy is very practical as well as spiritual.

## Nursing Staff

Nurses need the medical skills of symptom control, pain relief, and more, for each nurse is a teacher as well. Nurses assigned to a patient/family train the primary care person within that family in caring for the patient. This requires considerable skill, for the nurse (particularly in home care) may direct or assist in the patient's care, but encourages the primary care person to perform that care directly. Nurses are in close contact with the patient/family, and in the home-care setting may be the most frequently seen member of the team. Helping with the patient's care, visiting the family, and weathering the crises of terminal care together bring nurse and family close. The nurse is given many opportunities to assess the patient/family's needs and to communicate. The high level of interaction, plus the high level of nursing and communications skills required in terminal care, necessitate a high nurse-patient ratio—one nurse for each four patient/family units is desirable—so that hospices ideally budget 60 percent for personnel.

It may be that the best hospice nurse is an L.P.N.—licensed practical nurse—rather than an R.N. Today's R.N.s—registered nurses—are highly trained scientifically, and are sometimes reluctant to perform the more menial tasks necessary to keep a terminally ill patient comfortable. Preferring to use only those skills within an R.N.'s training (giving medications, for instance) can keep an R.N. from being a flexible hospice nurse. L.P.N.s also have a wide range of skills and are generally willing to do whatever the situation demands. This adaptability makes the L.P.N. very useful amid the changing events of terminal care. Needless to say, there are many R.N.s who are wonderful hospice nurses, but it would be advisable to have a large proportion of L.P.N.s on the staff as well. Reimbursement systems may make this difficult, however, as some sources will only pay for the services of an R.N. Restrictive third-party reimbursement may dictate staffing.

## Staff Stress

Staff "burnout" can be a hazard for anyone in the "helping" professions and for health-care workers particularly. Burnout causes withdrawal from patients, which is especially detrimental to hospice work. Team coordinators are aware of this and many of the programs that are basic for hospice work offset the staff stresses which can lead to burnout. In many ways, hospice is a less stressful environment than others in which death occurs. For example, there is no conflict between prolonging life and allowing death to occur, a frequent source of staff stress in an acute-care setting. Also, everyone on the staff is committed to hospice philosophy, which sees death as a natural occurrence and the comfort and peace of mind of the patient as the highest priorities. Staff assignments allow enough time to accomplish this and to allow for expressions of caring that are satisfying to patient and staff—time to sit and talk and listen. Positive relationships with patients, families, and other staff members, as well as positive community support and approval, compensate for the intensity of the work and ensure staff satisfaction. Flexible scheduling, which allows for time off and work rotation, also help.

The team structure has many built-in safeguards against burnout. The thorough orientation everyone receives inculcates a clear expectation of what the work will involve. In-service education keeps skills updated and can fill any needs for information the staff may have. Case management meetings allow for the contribution of each team member and also serve as a hospice review, ensuring that the program is meeting its goals for each patient/ family. Staff support meetings are also important and strengthen the interaction of team members. The patient and family need support and so does the staff.

## Patient and Staff Perceptions of Good Care

It is interesting to compare patient, family, and staff perceptions of the qualities needed by a care giver. Neal, White, and Buell surveyed terminally ill patients, their families, bereaved families, and staff (including the administrator) in ten hospice, hospital, nursing home, and home-care programs.[1] Among aspects of good care, a caring and compassionate staff was specified most frequently by patients. Patients also mentioned the importance of individualizing care, but this was secondary. Families of the dying stressed individualizing care most frequently, and secondly pain and symptom control and physical care, though they, too, mentioned a caring and compassionate staff. Like patients, bereaved families mentioned the desirability of a caring and compassionate staff most frequently. Individualizing patient care, and symptom control, as well as the understanding of the staff members, were also important. Families in both groups valued the availability of information and explanation. Staff members stressed individualizing patient care and family needs, and pain and symptom control. All groups basically agreed on what was important. Patients and families tended to speak of specific qualities appreciated in a care giver: friendliness, affection, and understanding. Staff tended to talk about qualities in broad terms, such as providing emotional support to patient/family.

There is another quality, not mentioned by the groups surveyed, which I believe to be important: humility. We "care givers" can become egotistical and overvalue our own importance. We forget how privileged we are to be able to serve and how much our patients give. As all of us know, egotism closes the heart and prevents real communication. Those who are close to death, and their families, teach and give so much, and we can receive their lessons best when our hearts are open. Those of us who work in a hospice situation are truly fortunate, for we have many opportunities to learn life's deepest lessons.

## Director of Volunteers

In addition to the medical director, the director of nurses, and the team coordinator, hospices need a director of volunteers, for volunteers play an exceedingly important role in hospice work. As I have discussed, volunteers must be screened in private interviews, trained, placed, and supported. Hospices usually do not receive reimbursement for volunteer services, yet volunteers enable hospice to offer a richer variety of programming than would otherwise be possible. The multidisciplinary team needs all its members.

## Appropriate Patient Referrals

It is important that physicians refer their terminally ill patients to a hospice when there is a prognosis of six months or less. Physicians are sometimes reluctant to make such a prognosis, fearing that the patient will be left without hope. Yet there are recognizable differences when a patient is in the terminal phase of an illness, and such a patient can benefit from palliative care. It has been recognized for a long time that for such a patient, further curative measures can unnecessarily prolong suffering and cause additional distress and exhaustion. Further tests and treatments upset the family also, when the patient's diagnosis is clearly established and he is fatigued by unnecessary procedures.

In order to maximize the benefits of hospice care, the patient should be referred early enough to benefit from hospice services. If referral is made several months before death, the patient and the family have time to finish any "business" they may have together and to renew their closeness as a family. The patient also has time to settle his affairs, and to grow from any lessons offered by his remaining time. These important concerns are more easily achieved with hospice support, practical measures for physical comfort, and the peaceful environment of the home or the hospice inpatient unit.

Physicians can learn to recognize when the terminally ill patient is within a few months of death, and can be educated to communicate this news gently, without instilling hopelessness. It is also important that the patient not be referred too early, when acute care is still appropriate. When treatment measures in an acute-care hospital have a chance of success, and the patient is still far from the terminal phase of illness, hospice is not the proper place for him. Aggressive treatment is best for a patient whose condition indicates hope for recovery. When cure is no longer possible and the patient is clearly in the terminal phase of disease, further aggressive therapy will only add to and prolong his suffering. It is then that the medical and humanistic palliative care of a hospice should be sought.

The cue, as always, must come from the patient. What are the patient's needs and preferences? Which services can best meet those needs? Patients are coming to think of themselves as medical-care consumers, with the right to choose the services that will benefit them most.

## Treatment of Nonphysical Needs

We have discussed palliative care and pain control for the patient's physical needs, but what about his emotional and spiritual needs? It is helpful for trained hospice staff to facilitate communication between patient and family, or just to sit and talk with the patient and allow him to express his thoughts and concerns. Psychiatry is not usually necessary. Dying is not necessarily an emotional or mental illness. It is an inevitable and a natural process which entails many changes and adjustments and which can lead to great individual growth before death. Professionals who can contribute to this growth are physical therapists, rehabilitation therapists, dance therapists, musicians, and members of the clergy.

The physical or rehabilitation therapist can be employed to maximize movement, and to help the patient use his physical resources most efficiently. Treatment is designed for this, and restoration of movement (in the curative sense) is not a goal. Dance therapists can help the patient to enjoy and retain a sense of pleasure in physical expression. Through gentle movement and exercise, a patient can keep some muscle tone for as long as possible. The bedbound patient may loose muscle prematurely through inactivity; with help he may be able to retain some strength for a longer period.

Creativity is a basic human need, which is shared by the terminally ill. Music, art, and creative writing can all help the patient to express thoughts and feelings, besides contributing to his enjoyment of life. Given peace of mind and physical comfort, a terminally ill person can often express great creativity. Perhaps the dying process itself forces reflection and introspection, which sometimes is manifested in beautiful poetry or drawing. Music can also be an outlet for this creativity, as well as a great pleasure. If the dying patient no longer has the strength to write, a poem, story, or song can be dictated to someone close. Sometimes these poems, songs, and observations of the dying possess a philosophical and spiritual tone.

## Hospice and Spirituality

A dying individual can hardly avoid spiritual questions, for the very process itself forces one to ask about the meaning of life and the eternal. Dying people sometimes describe experiences of love or of the spirit which help them prepare for the next stage of their journey. Whether or not the patient is formally religious, many of the dying feel a renewal of faith through their own experiences. Hospice staff (including a nondenominational chaplain) can support the patient's spiritual growth yet not intrude. Not all patients demonstrate this need, and their preferences must be respected. But for those patients who do seek spiritual answers, it is helpful to have a spiritually accepting and supportive environment. The willingness to talk about spiritual matters and the acknowledgment of a greater force than the visible, material world can contribute to the peace of mind of the dying patient.

St. Christopher's in London has many extended spiritual expressions, such as chapel services and communal hymns. American hospices may not wish to provide explicit expressions of religion, yet hospice by its very nature encompasses the spirit. In hospice philosophy, the human spirit is valued more and material things less. The motivation for the creation of hospices has been spiritual. Love and caring, and the peace of mind of the dying, are the goals, rather than a hospice's ability to create business profits. Even the attitude toward death is spiritual, for the individual's attitude of mind is more important than prolonging continuation in a material body. Many of the world's greatest spiritual scriptures have dealt with the question of death and have seen death as part of the soul's journey back to God. In the East, the dying person's state of mind at death is of major importance for the spiritual progress of that soul. During a terminal illness, the outward personality is often stripped away, revealing the spirit, or the person's deeper self. As one dying boy told his mother, "My real self is coming out with this illness."

Whether or not hospice professionals believe in God, or any particular religion, individual growth as part of the process of dying has often been observed. Dr. Lamerton of St. Joseph's Hospice in England said: "Dying is still a part of living. In this period a man may learn some of his life's most important lessons."[2] Elisabeth Kübler-Ross has given us many instances of this through her writing, her interviews with dying patients, and her reports of caring for them.

Hospice has its roots in the religious orders of the Christian Middle Ages, and until recent times hospices have been connected with religious orders. Though secular today, the hospice movement has been what Sandol Stoddard calls "faith in action." As she says: "Faith is the heart of this process and this profession, simply because there is no other force (by whatever name) that could cause people to behave toward one another as they do in the hospice situation."[3]

Though its roots are in ancient religious orders, and its motivation is spiritual, in matters of practical care hospice is very scientific. Perhaps there is no gap here at all. It may be as in modern physicists' talk of the unreality of matter and the reality of energy, science and spirituality echoing each other.

## Reimbursement

Though the loftiest goals of hospice soar to the heavens, it is rooted to the material plane; one does not exist without the other. Financial matters and reimbursement are necessarily of much concern. Hospice funding comes from a variety of sources: individuals and foundations, third-party payers (private carriers, Medicare, Medicaid, state and local government), and donations from such groups as United Way. As was mentioned earlier, the government recognizes the value of hospice both for humanitarian reasons and for practical ones; hospice care for the terminally ill is less expensive than acute-care hospitals. Legislation makes it possible for hospice programs to receive reimbursement from Medicare. Yet many services are not covered by either Medicare or insurance. Those services not covered include physician home visits, bereavement services, volunteer director services, homemaker services, and education services.[4] Also, many insurance companies fund only aggressive treatment rather than extended palliative care. There are many terminally ill patients who are too young for Medicare and are not eligible for other programs.

In this country, we have a tendency to fund institutional rather than home care, even though home care may be less expensive and more congenial. Medicaid, a state-run program, can fund home-care services for the elderly, but few states exercise that option. A further example of this bias is that nursing home benefits are more generous and consume more than 40 percent of the Medicaid budget, though alternatives are often less expensive.[5] Though Congress is working on legislation to fund more home-care programs, institutional care still receives the greatest reimbursement.

The institutionally based hospice does not have the financial difficulties of the independent hospice, but usually does not offer as great a variety of social services. Financial considerations may compel many hospice programs to seek shelter with an institution and may affect other hospice decisions as well. Funding may require a particular staff composition, R.N.s rather than L.P.N.s, for example.

## Institutionally Based Hospices Compared with Independent Hospices

Institutionally based hospices are often excellent due to the dedication of the medical directors and other staff, but there are some matters that trouble those who are involved in hospice development. Hospices housed in acute-care hospitals have significantly higher rates of institutional deaths than home-care hospices with inpatient backup. Patients of a hospital-based hospice unit die more frequently in the inpatient unit than at home. Home-care programs in these settings must be strengthened to be sure that patients receive a real choice. The institutional setting can become self-perpetuating, and administrators of such affiliated hospices must be sure that patients are not institutionalized unnecessarily. Hospice inpatient units must serve as backup for home-care patients. Ideally, even if the inpatient unit is necessary temporarily, with additional support the patient may be able to return home. In other words, institutionalization should not be a permanent solution for most hospice patients. Independent hospices with inpatient backup units have stronger home-care programs and a record of more patients cared for and dying at home. There is concern that higher rates of institutional deaths in institutionally based hospices reflect a loss of hospice philosophy. If we are not vigilant about maintaining hospice standards of care, we could end up right where we started, with inappropriate care for the terminally ill.

Hospital administrators feel financial pressure to fill empty beds and it may be that this pressure extends to hospices in hospitals. There may also be a temptation to fill beds in other hospital areas with "hospice" patients, and hospice medical directors may find themselves struggling to maintain the psychological and physical environment necessary for hospice patients. The results may be unsatisfactory for patient, for medical director, and for hospital administration as well. Institutional hospices are surrounded by an atmosphere of urgency, haste, and machinery in the acute-care setting.

Sir Michael Sobell House in Oxford, England, is a hospice with a separate unit though it is located on the grounds of Churchill Hospital. Sandol Stoddard describes this hospice as homey and cozy, with the characteristics of a small community. Children are welcomed with treats and decorations designed for them. Stoddard says: "Everything about the unit suggests medical expertise, yet nothing here is strange, forbidding, or frightening."[6]

Hospices within a hospital do not have as much freedom to create a homey environment, and usually do not have as much space as an independent hospice. The play schools one sees at St. Christopher's, or at Hospice, Inc., in Branford, Connecticut, are absent. The atmosphere and visiting hours are more likely to be restrictive for children. Hospices within an institution have a more hospital-like environment, although the care for terminally ill patients is superior to the hospital's and more personalized. Institutionally based hospices hope that the hospital climate will be modified and improved as other areas of the hospital see the success of hospice methods. Hospices within institutions may serve as models and teachers if care is taken to adhere to hospice philosophy.

## Hospital Care

There are times, as I have said, when an acute-care hospital is the appropriate place for a patient. Modern medical technology can cure many illnesses, and so long as the patient's condition indicates the possibility of cure, then the hospital is the place for him or her. Even when this is not the case, some patients, or their families (such as the Ziccarelli family in Chapter 2), wish to continue with aggressive treatment until the end. Their wishes must be respected and for them the hospital is the best choice.

There are also situations in which financial considerations and other factors make the hospital the best choice, as is the case with my friend Henry. Henry is a Mexican-American, sixty-two years old, dying of cancer of the larynx which has spread throughout his body. Large tumors fill his throat and make speech impossible. Henry must breathe with a hole in the front of his neck.

Henry qualifies for hospice care and would like to die at home very much. Unfortunately, there is no one to take care of him. His mother is eighty-five and barely able to care for herself. Henry's ex-wife loves him and visits daily, but her mental problems (she has been diagnosed as a paranoid schizophrenic) leave her unable to care for him; indeed, she, too, has difficulty caring for herself. Their only child is a fifteen-year-old girl, who has been sent to boarding school under the sponsorship of a rich relative. There is no primary care person for Henry.

Cost is a problem for him and he could not afford inpatient hospice care without help. Since he is a veteran, there is no charge for him at the Veterans Hospital, so there he is.

The Veterans Hospital is giving him excellent, compassionate care. Traditional therapy is done for symptom relief, and the staff understands and has training in palliative care. Nurses and aides make sure that Henry is comfortable and that pain and other symptoms are under control. Henry feels that he is getting good care, but he is bored and lonely.

When, during our last visit, I asked how he felt, Henry wrote me a note, with difficulty: "I feel trapped, no place to go." He is in a room by himself and cannot talk to anyone. His friends no longer visit because they are afraid of death and of someone close to death. Henry was always a sociable, active man and this is hard on him. He worked all his life out in the sunshine as a mason (including on my house) and it is difficult for him to be indoors all the time.

I spoke to some of the staff about Henry's nonphysical needs and they promised some roommates the next day. An orderly now takes Henry for rides in his wheelchair outdoors, so Henry can visit the hospital's lovely grounds. Henry needs activity and the occupational therapist visits with things for him to do. So in the midst of a modern hospital, Henry is dying with attention to all his needs. He will retain his individuality to the end of his life.

## Edifice Complex

Hospice home-care programs can exist without an institution. We must not obscure our vision of hospice with buildings, or develop an "edifice" complex. Inpatient units are helpful as backup for the home-care program, and offer an alternative for some patients, but a hospice program can begin without a building. Hospice is an attitude toward life and toward death; it is an attitude of caring, of personal treatment that values the human spirit and sees each human being as worthy of love and care, regardless of his or her age or physical condition. Hospice sees the patient as giver as well as receiver. Hospice is more than a building, though buildings help facilitate hospice services. Hospice is a philosophy and practice of care.

## Evaluation of Hospice Programs

Further evaluations of hospice home-care programs are necessary, as are evaluations of terminal care, which has been insufficiently assessed. Hospice program evaluation is essential to provide the rationale for decisionmaking, to clarify the direction of future programming, and to supply the incentive to institute needed corrective measures. Appraisal of the degree to which programs meet the goals they were established and contracted to achieve is a necessary prerequisite for the extension of the hospice concept throughout the country.

Pressure for greater accountability will be placed upon hospice as it moves into the sphere of broad-range, country-wide community service. The faith of the public it is to serve is fundamental to the program's universal establishment. Evaluations of both home-care and inpatient hospice programs will help create the yard-sticks by which one may measure standards of success, so that criteria may be validated and new criteria of effectiveness developed. Knowledge of the usefulness of specific procedures or techniques may help to identify logical applications of further efforts; advancing knowledge will affect assumptions, goals, and activities. In directing the course of future efforts in the field of terminal care, evaluations of the effectiveness of hospice care can increase the efficacy of innovative programs, point up areas requiring further research, and suggest possible alternatives to be explored. In the light of research findings, more desirable means for attaining the designated objectives may be proposed. It is vital to determine whether and how well hospice objectives are being met, and to ascertain the causes of specific successes or failures.

Evaluation studies and standards of care may help with reimbursement of a greater variety of hospice services. The government now acknowledges the value and cost efficiency of hospice programs, and more funding may become available. Funding is especially needed for home-care programs and for extended care for the terminally ill in every age bracket. Though home and hospice care is considerably less expensive than standard acute care in hospitals, some families may suffer financially when insurance companies reimburse only aggressive treatment. Perhaps insurance companies will offer their policyholders more options to cover these realities in the future. I hope that both public and private funding and reimbursement will help families care for their relative at home if they wish, and will help inpatient hospice units to realize the highest ideals of care.

## Choosing a Hospice

In choosing a hospice program what are the qualities to look for? Here is a list of some basic characteristics:

- *The Hospice Program:* Home care should be the heart of the program, with coordinated inpatient backup if necessary. The program should also be autonomous, with freedom to make decisions whether or not the program is independent or housed within an acute-care facility.
- *Primary unit of care:* Patient and family.
- *Symptom control:* The hospice staff should be knowledgeable about the medical control of all physical symptoms. There should be attention also to the patient's nonphysical needs—emotional, social, and spiritual.
- *Medical director:* A physician or nurse with a sound professional background should be the medical director. A group of well-meaning people alone cannot make a hospice.
- *Multidisciplinary team:* Hospice services should be coordinated by a multidisciplinary team including social worker, physical and occupational therapist, pastoral care, and consultant services as needed. The family and volunteers are also part of the team.
- *Volunteers:* Trained selected volunteers help the hospice provide a wider variety of services.
- *Services available on call:* Hospice services must be available seven days a week, twenty-four hours a day.
- *Bereavement follow-up:* Depending upon the needs of the individual family, these services will vary, but they should be available.

- *Hospice education:* Ideally, hospices have education programs available to the community.
- *Services based on need:* Hospice services should be based on need rather than ability to pay.

When looking at an inpatient hospice, note the interaction between patients and staff (smiles, relaxed manner, personal interest and concern, etc.), the general atmosphere (cheerful, noninstitutional-looking), and the provisions for families and children. Can families stay overnight if they wish? Can relatives cook a special meal? Is there a place for children to play? Are there open (unrestricted) visiting hours?

If you or someone in your family needs a hospice, then you are on a very special journey together, and will want a hospice that lives up to all the ideals described in this book.

## Hospice and the Community

Hospices throughout this country and in England have begun as local community efforts. Small groups of people—medical professionals, clergy, and concerned citizens—begin to meet, do research, and plan a hospice in their community. Next, a small grant or donation makes it possible to hire a staff member or to rent a small office (as in Hospice, Inc., in Branford). Sometimes the hospice begins as an office in someone's home (as in Hospice Orlando), able to offer a home-care program because of the volunteer efforts of a physician and nurses. Community support increases as friends and neighbors of patients hear about a patient's relief from pain and distress, and some give donations in gratitude or become volunteers. Hospice has truly been a grass-roots movement of loving service with the community.

## Public Relations and Information

Individual hospices have had small community beginnings, but each hospice has had to establish relations with the larger community. The public needs information about hospice, about what hospice does and can do, about the attitudes toward life and death that make hospice work. Attitudes are changing, but a community may need further help, or society's general denial of death may lead to prejudice against the hospice concept. When a small and carefully organized group in New Haven began to search for a site for Hospice, Inc., community opposition in one town blocked settlement. Hospice, Inc., had to spend time preparing the community and educating possible neighbors before a site in Branford was agreed upon.

## Uncovering the Hidden Issue of Death

Ongoing public education about the doings of a local hospice increases community awareness. There have been many programs on television during the past few years which have increased public attention to the needs of the dying and the bereaved. Numerous books, magazine articles, and public lectures have also helped to sensitize people to the needs of the terminally ill. We have come a long way since Kübler-Ross began the patient interviews that became *On Death and Dying,* and have come to talk more about death, but we still have a way to go toward acceptance of death as a part of life. Visible hospices, or home-care hospice programs, help people see and accept that death is an inevitable part of life and should not be hidden away.

In the recent past (and even today), patients have been sent to the hospital just because they were dying, even if the hospital had nothing to offer them. We tend to isolate and ignore what frightens us, and we have been afraid of death. When home care takes place, neither the patient nor the family is isolated from the rest of the community, and death becomes a more naturally accepted event. Just as, in the hospice environment, we do not deny death, we do not deny the grief of the bereaved.

Hospice can contribute to public awareness and acceptance by continuing to be a community within the community. Adults who have contact with a hospice may have a deeper understanding of the dying and of death, and may see their own lives differently. Children also need such exposure, and may be taught from an early age that death is an expected and natural occurrence. The day-care centers on the grounds of St. Christopher's in London and Hospice, Inc., in Branford exist for the hospice staff and the children and grandchildren of the patients. These children bring vitality to hospice, and a sense of community with all the stages and ages of life, and in turn these children are given the gifts of compassion and learn that neither the old nor the terminally ill are frightening or foreign, but are simply their loving friends, grand-parents, or parents at the end of life. These interactions strengthen community awareness and acceptance and extend the hospitality of the hospice to all who enter its doors.

## Interagency Cooperation

As a part of the local community, hospice works with all other service groups in the area. Local groups may trade referrals and services and work together cooperatively. Visiting nurse associations can provide much support and many services to bedbound patients at home. Visiting nurses are usually available only during the day, Monday through Friday. Most hospice services are available twenty-four hours a day and on weekends. These two agencies can work together very harmoniously (as described in Chapter 2) for mutual benefits. Hospice planners must understand local needs and know which human-service agencies are in their area.

## Medical Fragmentation

Working cooperatively with other agencies in the area, and with the patient's personal physician, can reduce some of the fragmentation of medical services that most patients suffer through. Because each area of medical specialty works independently and there is no coordinator of health care, a patient and family may be sent from one doctor to another, from the intensive care unit to the coronary care unit or the oncology unit, and perhaps to the hospice unit. Fragmentation of services confuses and disturbs and needlessly harasses the patient, and is very expensive. This is the opposite of the caring community that is hospice, with its variety of skilled professionals who are part of one team. Because hospice care is so different in concept and practice from care the patient receives elsewhere, we must be careful not to let hospice become just another specialty, but must integrate its services with the rest of the community.

It is hoped that hospice care will become standard care in the years to come and will be given by all health-care personnel. Hospitality need not be only for the dying but, as in medieval times, for the woman in labor or the very ill as well. Most of the concepts of hospice work could very well apply to other health-care agencies: the multidisciplinary team, which sees to the needs of the family as well as the patient; personal care, which includes knowing the patient's name as well as his individual condition; attention to relief of symptoms as well as cure; an attitude toward human beings that sees every individual as worthy of loving care; and the acceptance of death as a natural occurrence. Concern and care can go very well with expert professional skills, and do in hospice. I sincerely hope, too, that the education of medical and nursing students everywhere will include hospice's concepts of care and its philosophy of humane treatment of the dying and their families.

Within hospice, prevention of fragmentation is achieved through the variety of skills and social services offered. Counseling is available for patient and family if needed; financial planning and help with making out a will are also available. Volunteers help the home-care patient with transportation, with homemaking, with children, and perform a variety of other services. Physicians, nurses, and therapists notice the patient's changing conditions and prevent difficulties wherever possible. The patient's social and spiritual needs are given attention as well. Less urgent needs are also considered, and some hospices have beauty salon equipment and have found volunteers with hairdressing skills. All these skilled people work together, not only as a team but as a community.

## Regulation

Regulation is an essential factor in any skilled profession. The hospice medical staff must be expert in their craft and have thorough knowledge of the newer methods of pain and symptom control. Particular emphasis is placed on the art of medicine, but the craft is essential too. Pharmacologists must be knowledgeable and competent. Besides sympathy and friendly communication and teaching, the nurses give highly skilled care. A group of well-meaning people without these skills cannot make up a hospice. There must be *uniform standards* of care before the name hospice can be used. As Sandol Stoddard says: "Groups or individuals promising to provide 'an easy death' by removing the patient from medical professionals and performing some sort of hocus-pocus with or without the use of drugs are so far from being hospices that it is hard to imagine them trying to use the name; but there are reasons to believe that some will, and they should be guarded against." [7]

Hospice is becoming a popular idea which may tempt some to imitate superficial features of the concept without providing actual hospice care. I feel strongly that this would weaken the whole hospice movement and damage its credibility with the public as well as possible sources of reimbursement. Agencies using the name without the meaning behind it would hurt the very people hospice is most concerned about—the patient and the family. Patients and families need information about hospice standards of care and what services they may expect. Further evaluations of present hospices can establish these standards and provide models for future hospices.

## Popularity: Help or Hazard?

Since the humble beginnings of the first American hospice home-care program, in New Haven in 1974, hospices have been established in many communities throughout the country, and many more are in various stages of development. Hospice is a popular idea, and those who are involved in the movement are pleased to see its acceptance. It is encouraging to see how many hospices have been developed under the leadership of physicians and nurses, who are changing traditional medical practice. However, overpopularity has it dangers. Hospice concepts are endorsed by both conservative and liberal politicians, by both young and old, and this is as it should be; but could hospice become a cliché like motherhood and apple pie, receiving sentimental endorsement without much thought for the underlying philosophy? Popularity can also lead to smugness and complacency, which in turn lead to stagnation. Hospice must continue to meet the needs of those it aims to serve, humbly and flexibly. Hospice needs more than sentimental support, just as the dying do; both need a heartfelt commitment as well as realistic and practical aid.

Hospice has survived the centuries; it has survived neglect and abandonment and will survive popularity. Perhaps hospice procedures and attitudes will become standard medical care in the years to come, both in private practice and in acute-care hospitals. Perhaps "hospice" and "hospital" will once again have the same meaning, as they did centuries ago.

# 4 ❦
# Costs of Hospice Care

There is an urgent need for more explicit information concerning the type, length, and cost of hospice care. Hospice has succeeded in its aim to decrease the cost of care to patients and their families. The proof of this is the major legislation passed by Congress in July 1982, and signed by President Reagan, that includes hospice care as a federally reimbursable program. However, we must realize that the cost of hospice care cannot be measured just in dollars and cents.

Hospice care acknowledges the cost of commitment—that is, the emotional, social, and psychological cost to the patient and to the patient's family. Often these costs, which continue after the death of the patient, are the greatest. To date, they have not been adequately measured.

When a loved one dies, for example, there is often an increase in the use of barbiturates and alcohol by the bereaved. Sometimes family members continue their use dangerously until an addictive problem arises. Certainly this cost is difficult to measure. And it may be more expensive than all the dollar costs of physical care. Other costs may include the number of workdays lost by both patient and family members and resultant loss of income. There are the hidden costs of family disruption following a death, and an increased divorce rate among parents who have lost a child.

Though the hospice movement in the United States has made definite inroads into the established health-care delivery system within the last decade, there is still significant reluctance by the establishment to accept the hospice concept of health care as a viable option in standard patient-care procedures. Three major concerns need to be addressed before hospice care is accepted by health-care practitioners, third-party payers, and the general public: defining and determining a market for hospice care; demonstrating cost effectiveness of hospice care compared to current standard health-care procedures; and assuring third-party reimbursement for hospice care.

A study of St. Mary's Hospital in Richmond, Virginia, found that cancer patients compose a reasonable sample of hospice-care candidates. "Of 245 persons identified as being potential hospice candidates, 239 (97.5%) were cancer patients."[1] (Hospice candidates were defined as those dying of chronic terminal illness and living within the primary service area of the hospital. For further analysis, please see Appendix B, Characteristics of Cancer Patients Identified.) The majority of these hospice-care candidates were over sixty years old and the most frequently occurring time interval between initial diagnosis and death was seven to twenty-four months.

Another area of concern in determining a hospice market is public awareness and acceptance of the hospice concept of health care. A study utilizing 203 adult respondents in the tricounty area of metropolitan Detroit revealed the following: three-quarters of the respondents had never heard of hospice; of those who did, the majority said they did not understand it.

Following an educational module on hospice:

- Ninety-two percent claimed to understand it (verified by a written explanation).
- A large majority viewed hospice care as being different from hospital care for the terminally ill.
- Nearly all the participants said they considered hospice the preferred way to care for the dying.
- Two-thirds would choose hospice care for themselves.
- One-third were still unsure.[2]

Finally, this study identified eight major concerns expressed by the respondents about hospice care:

- The extent to which families would be allowed to be involved in the patient's care.
- Possible interferences with personal and family freedoms.
- Sufficient personnel being available to give adequate support to the patient and his family.
- Commitment of personnel to the special quality of care needed by the dying patient.
- Availability and accessibility of hospice services.
- The cost of hospice services.
- Comfort and pain control.
- Remaining alert and functioning while undergoing treatment.[3]

While these concerns are legitimate, the hospice concept addresses each one of them directly and specifically.

The market for hospice care as defined and determined by these studies is extremely viable. In relating hospice's future to the total health-care market, it is important to note that we are an increasingly long-lived society. Also, a significant number of Americans develop cancer each year. (For statistics on life expectancy and on the incidence of cancer in our population, see Appendix C. Charts showing the percentage of U.S. population aged sixty-five and older by region and state, and the leading causes of death by region, can be found in Appendixes D and E).

The next area of concern for hospice care is that of demonstrating cost effectiveness compared with standard available procedures. Several recent studies have compared the costs of hospice treatment with those of nursing homes and hospitals.

One study analyzed costs of a home-care hospice—Hospice of Columbus (Ohio)—compared to costs of similar nursing home and hospital services. The total hospice budget was approximately $522 per day. If these costs had been distributed among patients for payment, they would have averaged $65 per day. Staff salaries, when averaged among patients, were $45 per day—$25 for nursing salaries and $20 for administrative salaries.

The study then compared costs of home-care hospice, hospital, and skilled nursing home. Hospital care in the same community would have averaged $126 per day; nursing-home care, $50 per day. Thus, forty-two days of hospice care would have cost about the same as twenty-two days in a hospital. Charges for a physician or for medication would have been an added expense in all the situations (home-care hospice, hospital, and nursing home). Hospice care averaged $15 more per day than the nursing home. Hospice care is likely to become more competitive with nursing-home costs as hospice becomes more efficient with experience. As the volunteer program is strengthened, the services they provide will increase efficiency and lower costs.[4] (For more detail on this study, see Appendix F.)

Another recent study analyzing comparative costs of treatment practices for the terminally ill uses data from Hospice, Inc., New Haven, to illustrate the premise that the cost of hospice outpatient care of terminally ill patients is only 10 percent to 20 percent of the cost of chronic hospitalization.

It was found that the average length of stay in the Connecticut hospice program was seventy-six days per patient. Statistics collected on the number and duration of home visits by staff members reveal that in a smoothly running hospice program, the nurse visits every four to five days; the physician visits about once a month; the social worker once during the patient's care; and the pastoral-care person less than that. (These are averages; individual families and patients may need more or less from different staff members.) It was also interesting to find that these home visits were of a longer average time than many patients have with health-care professionals in other settings. For example, the doctor usually visited around forty-seven minutes (an unusual length of time for many physicians), the nurse usually stayed for over an hour, while the social worker visited for about an hour and a half. The total cost of seventy-six days in the hospice program averaged $1,320. A hospital stay for the same length of time would have been considerably higher.[5]

A third study, funded by Blue Cross and Blue Shield, utilized terminally ill patients treated by the Genesee Region Home Care

Association in New York. The total cost of care provided by this organization equaled $118,626 for 1,576 days of patient care provided to the fifty-five patients in the study. If the patients had not received the home hospice services, their physicians estimated, 943 days of hospital care would have been required, at a cost of $212,175. The savings amounts to $93,549.[6]

Finally, the most convincing cost analysis research studied nineteen matched pairs of terminally ill patients treated in a home or a hospital setting during the final two weeks of life. (See Appendixes G and H.) The most striking conclusion of this study is that hospital treatment for the last two weeks of life is 10.5 times greater in costs than home care. According to the researchers, the tenfold increase bought more intensive technological measures and diagnostic, therapeutic, and palliative treatment. The cost of palliation for those at home was $70, compared to $1,763 at the hospital.[7]

These four studies provide convincing evidence of the magnitude of cost variation between hospice and chronic-care facilities in treating the terminally ill. They consistently conclude that hospice care is far less costly than chronic-care hospitalization.

The last major area to be discussed in relation to the proliferation of hospice care is third-party reimbursement. Because of new concepts fundamental to hospice care (bereavement visits, respite care, support services for family members, etc.), third-party payers have shown a reluctance to fund hospice treatment in its entirety.

In deciding whether hospice care should be reimbursed, the following three principles, proposed by Blue Cross and Blue Shield in 1978, must be followed:

- There must be demonstrated community need for hospice services or programs.
- There must be assurances that the care provided meets medically acceptable standards of health-care administration.
- There must be assurances that the delivery of hospice care is performed in an efficient and economical manner and physical setting that make effective use of existing community resources.[8]

The recommendations from Blue Cross and Blue Shield refer both to the hospice program and to payment. Program recommendations emphasize that the care offered should include both home care and inpatient services. Only after the patient satisfied specific criteria regarding condition, prognosis, and home and family conditions would he/she be eligible. Blue Cross and Blue Shield wish to ascertain that hospice programs will work with already existing health-care providers, to be sure that all the care a patient needs will be available. They also request means of determining whether hospice care is necessary or appropriate for the patient. Lastly, hospice programs will need to comply with local and state health regulations and with any accreditation requirements.

Initial payments from Blue Cross and Blue Shield will be on a demonstration basis, to be followed with an evaluation. Existing benefit provisions will be followed whenever possible, though there will be some flexibility. Payments will be made only where patient and services meet specific criteria, and where care is given effectively and economically. Costs are not to exceed charges for care in traditional settings.[9]

Because a great deal of evidence has been gathered to satisfy the concerns of third-party payers in recent years, increasing reimbursement of hospice care will make hospice treatments a viable alternative to the standard chronic-care hospitalization of the terminally ill. A substantial savings in cost to the whole society would result, since 80 percent of the population die in chronic-care facilities.[10]

Inherent in hospice are many costs and benefits that do not readily facilitate the assignment of a dollar value. These relate to both the patient and his family.

Treated in a hospital, the patient gives up much of his right of self-determination. Hospitals are institutions, where patients are categorized and assigned according to their condition and immediate prognosis. Such an environment tends to exacerbate the feelings of "contamination" that cancer patients often have. Nursing procedures may contribute to these feelings. Standard attention to

sanitary practices may be translated by the patient as being directly related to his medical condition. Because medical intervention
is limited for the terminally ill patient, physician visits are often
short and have little tangible value from the patient's point of
view. Having little to offer to the patient from a medical standpoint, physicians tend to delegate more time to other, nonterminal
patients, for whom medical intervention has some visible and gratifying result.

As for the family, visits to a patient in a hospital are often highly
ritualized. Family members and patient assume standardized roles
of behavior. Meaningful personal exchange is handicapped by in-
terruptions from the hospital staff and consideration for other patients. A frequent problem for treatment of the terminally ill in
hospitals is the often haphazard assignment of "roommates."
What kind of psychological implications arise in the terminally ill
patient when his roommate is recovering from an acute condition?
Obviously the doctor pays more visits and spends more time with
a patient whose prognosis is gratifying. Also, the hospital staff tend
to give more attention to someone who is recovering, out of reluctance to face death and the dying process. Can the hospital staff
handle the concerns and questions of a dying patient? Can they
handle the frequent question: "How much longer must I go
through this?" Since most people in a hospital are not there with a
terminal illness, the hospital staff may not be experienced in handling such a "defeatist" concept as dying or acceptance of death.

Hospice care, on the other hand, deals directly with the concerns of the terminally ill, so that the special considerations of
terminal care are addressed. In addition, there are special considerations, which often are overlooked. Treated in a home hospice
setting, the patient is part of the total home environment, able to
witness and often to participate in real-life events—meal-making,
family discussions, and other daily routines. This provides a vital
link with life. Seeing that life is a continuous, ongoing process
provides some comfort to the patient facing death. Also, the home
provides a setting more congenial to intimacy with family members and hospice staff.

Several eventualities must be considered before home hospice care is selected by the patient and his family as the course of treatment. One is the loss of wages by family members who take time off from work to care for the patient. Furthermore, involvement in the treatment of the dying is emotionally draining and often exceedingly traumatic. Family members may face ethical decisions in regard to the patient's care. For example, should oxygen be given in the final stages of the disease when breathing becomes irregular and shallow, or should "natural" events be allowed to follow their course? Finally, the moment of death and its aftermath may be traumatic. The body of a loved one turning dark from lack of oxygen may recur in the mind of the survivors long after the patient has died.

Once these situations are addressed by the care givers and accepted, home hospice care provides valuable spiritual and psychological benefits. Witnessing the death of a loved one enables us more easily to handle our own inevitable mortality. Also, special insights and intimate thoughts are shared in the relationship between dying person and survivors. As one saying goes, you can know how a person lived by how he or she dies. From a psychological standpoint, home hospice care provides an opportunity to avoid later feelings of guilt. The family members as care givers are comforted in the knowledge that they were directly involved in attending to their loved one in a time of greatest need. Family members' presence during the final moments of the patient's life afford a peaceful and tranquil end, with people who genuinely care. At this time, family members are together in an environment where they can immediately express their thoughts and feelings among one another, which sets up a framework for mutual support during the bereavement process.

Hospice care, then, demonstrates through both tangible and intangible costs and benefits its viability as an alternative to the chronic-care institutionalization of the terminally ill. However, for hospice care to be a widely used resource, its proponents must deal with our society's negative feelings toward death and dying. For people have learned to avoid the reality of the dying process by placing the terminally ill in chronic-care institutions and then letting hospital and funeral directors care for them. The result is guilt and an absence of deep and significant human relationships throughout all life's stages, one of which is death.

# 5 ❧
# Hospice Programs
# and Dying Children

Hospice programs in the United States and Europe have addressed the needs of the terminally ill adult and geriatric patient very well, and attention is now turning to the terminally ill child, from birth through eighteen years of age. The National Hospice Organization reports that there are now eight hundred programs in the United States offering some form of hospice care, yet fewer than twenty of these offer services for children. Visiting nurse associations do not always have pediatric programs either, even in large cities with nearby pediatric oncology and cystic fibrosis centers.

Why are there so few programs for the care of dying children other than acute-care hospitals? Is there a need for such programming? We will address some of these questions in this chapter, as well as the particular needs of dying children and their families. We will also discuss home-care programs for terminally ill children, and the benefits for the family. Other relevant hospice services will be examined, such as day programs and inpatient units. Reimbursement reflects the difference in perception of needs for ill children and adults, as aggressive treatment is more likely to receive funds than palliative care, another important problem. Differences and similarities between terminally ill children and adults are also of interest.

This chapter was written by Robert W. Buckingham and Leah Loveday.

Cancer is now the major cause of death by disease in children and teens, with 1 in 10,000 children under age eighteen stricken—approximately 6,000 children diagnosed annually.[1] While these figures are high compared with other life-threatening childhood diseases, they are low when compared with the incidence of cancer in adults, which is ten times greater. The most common childhood cancer is acute lymphocytic leukemia, with 2,500 new cases in children reported every year. Today, about half the children with this disease are able to stay in remission for five years, and of those who do, 85 percent may be able to recover completely. Other childhood cancers, such as Wilms's tumor, also have high survival rates. Children frequently contract different forms of cancer than are seen in adults. Neuroblastoma (tumors which begin in young nerve cells) is found only in children, three-quarters of the victims showing symptoms before age five. Though the survival rate is hopeful for some forms of cancer prevalent among children, many of these cancers are incurable and claim about 2,000 children a year. Relapses extend the process, with the child requiring care for a number of years (three to five, with leukemia).

There are also a number of other illnesses that afflict children, such as cystic fibrosis, heart defects, and kidney disorders, which claim many young lives. These are slow diseases, for the most part, with a terminal phase which may last for several months (just as with adults) and may cause pain and multiple discomforts.

Children suffer just as adults do from the physical stress of dying and have many of the same emotional and spiritual needs as the adult patient. The child's family, of course, suffers considerable stress and disruption. Both need long-term support—social, physical, emotional, psychological, and spiritual.

With all the potential benefits for a child and family from hospice care, why are there so few programs for terminally ill children? Part of the answer might be that it is so hard for parents and doctors to admit that the child is terminally ill. As the director of a children's hospice program (still in the planning stage) said recently: "Everyone looks so hard for remission that the child might be dying while receiving aggressive therapy." It is often difficult to accept death as a natural occurrence in an acute-care setting, and the feeling that death is unnatural is even stronger when the patient is a child. Nurses and other medical personnel, shaken by tending to someone "too young to die," are tempted to hide their feelings. The child's doctor may have a particularly hard time, for he has usually treated the child over a number of years, and may feel a personal investment in prolonging the child's life. The physician may see the death of a young patient as a failure, a personal failure as well as a failure of the medical system, and may react by abandoning the terminally ill child and the family or continuing efforts for a cure.

It is particularly difficult in our time to accept the death of a young person. The increase in longevity has caused us to equate death with old age, and to think of death as a remote prospect. We place a high value on youth and childhood in our country, and an early death is seen as occurring out of phase, unnatural. The death rates for children have decreased dramatically since the beginning of this century, from over 1,000 deaths per 100,000 population in 1900 to slightly less than 60 deaths per 100,000 population in 1967 in children from one to four years of age. (See Appendix I.) Early deaths are seen as a high social loss, and we mourn the young person's potential as well as the present tragedy. Also, the vast growth in scientific knowledge and medical technology in this century has led to the near elimination of many formerly fatal childhood diseases, and to the expectation that all diseases can be eliminated, that death itself can be "cured." We value our children so highly that it is particularly difficult for us to allow them to die, forgoing aggressive attempts at treatment for the gentler methods of palliative care. Physicians, nurses, and parents make great efforts to cure, and when these efforts are unsuccessful are all the more reluctant to recognize the terminal phase of the child's illness.

Perhaps giving a prognosis of six months or less for a child with a life-threatening disease represents an admission we resist making. Perhaps pity for the child (and the parents) prevents us from seeing the child's real needs and attending to them. Terminally ill children, like adults, deserve our compassion and empathy rather than our pity, deserve our best efforts for their comfort and peace of mind.

As hospice workers have found with adults, the family and patient must be the unit of care. Parents of a terminally ill child suffer greatly and need the concerned support of a team that understands their emotional, psychological, and physical needs. The diagnosis itself, even when suspected, is often a great shock to families, and may sometimes be seen by parents of a deceased child as an even greater stress than the death.[2] Relapses after remission, for parents of a child with cancer, are a renewed source of anxiety, and the strain of an uncertain future exacts its toll on the health and mental well-being of the family. Each remission, each hospitalization, is a reminder that the disease may become terminal. Most parents continue to hope until the disease becomes far advanced. Many adopt a style of "crisis coping," spending their time and energies on the sick child, learning about the disease and various treatments, and coping with emergencies while other personal and family matters are kept pending. If the child is hospitalized, both parents may take time off from work, or alternate so that someone is with the child, while siblings are placed with relatives or friends.

Many children are taken to major treatment centers (oncology or cystic fibrosis) in their state, which are frequently far from home. This adds to the financial and emotional stress of the family, and separates its members, for the mother usually moves to be near the child while the father continues to work and care for other siblings. If there is a nearby Ronald McDonald House the family is fortunate, for then they can all afford to stay together in a homey environment and meet other families in the same situation, offering mutual support. Ronald McDonald Houses throughout the country are locally owned and staffed temporary homes for the families of children being treated for life-threatening illnesses. They are particularly helpful when parents have to commute some distance to the hospital or treatment center and would otherwise spend the night in the hospital, dozing in the lobby or on a cot to be near their child. Ronald McDonald Houses are usually close to the hospital, frequently within walking distance. Sometimes the child can be treated as an outpatient and stay with his/her family in the nearby Ronald McDonald House. Though a nominal fee is requested when the family can afford it, expensive motel bills, which add to the great financial burden of treatment, are avoided.

Amid the family stress, it is possible to overlook the central figure, the patient. The patient needs information, yet parents of a child with a fatal illness generally experience great difficulty in communicating openly with him or her. They wonder how much the child knows or should know about the diagnosis and prognosis. We tend to protect children, and formerly believed that children could not comprehend death, and would not be able to understand the meaning of their illness or deal with the prospects emotionally if told. Research has shown that children comprehend the seriousness of their disease without being told directly. Even a two-year-old may understand and be aware of impending death. A mother told one of the authors that her two-and-a-half-year-old daughter knew of her relapse before the tumor was revealed with tests, and said her "owie came back." She wanted to "go home," by which she clearly did not mean her parents' house. Kübler-Ross has shown in her work with children that drawings done by even a very young terminally ill child can reveal the child's inner knowledge in symbolic form. Since the child does have a very clear idea of the fate that approaches, the need for open communication is all the greater. The young patient who is denied discussion of the seriousness of his illness may feel isolated, or believe that others are not aware of what he is experiencing. Children often protect their parents and will not discuss taboo topics.

Whether or not the child expresses a need for discussion, he particularly needs his parents' support at this time and is especially sensitive to them. If he is not allowed to express freely his own reaction to his illness and prognosis, he may feel cut off from his parents. Difficult as it is, the parents need to include the child in discussion of the diagnosis and possible treatments so that they may share their doubts and concerns. One small boy demonstrated his need by carefully hiding a box with all his photos which he had removed from the family album. "It was his way of making a statement about his parents' refusal to talk to him about his disease and his way of acknowledging that he might no longer be part of the family. 'We were no longer separate,' his mother recalled later (after discovering the child with his box). 'He was only four, too young to be troubled, I thought.' Now Jeff and his mother could comfort each other with the knowledge that they weren't suffering alone."[3]

Children who know that their parents do not wish to talk about their cancer may appear unconcerned, but their drawings reveal their insight. "One father emphatically did not want his child to be told he had cancer, and once a week in the clinic his child always drew his father without ears."[4] One mother found that she and her twelve-year-old son were able to become much closer when they could discuss his impending death. The boy took the lead by saying, "I wouldn't mind dying, but you'd mind, wouldn't you?" After initial resistance, and work on her own fears, this mother was able to reopen the topic and leave it open between them. The boy revealed his own fears, not of death—"I'm not afraid to die," he said—but that "everyone will be sad." "Mom will be sad," he anxiously told a hospice-trained nurse. Mother and son had many talks, and he was able to accept her sadness and know that she would be all right, just as he was. His remaining months were spent in great peace.

In a desire to protect children from the reality of their condition, we actually increase their burdens. As Myra Bluebond-Langer found in her work with victims of leukemia, terminally ill children of all ages come to know that they are dying. However, when parents or other adults avoid the topic, the child must pretend ignorance. She advocates allowing the child to communicate openly with those who can handle it, and to practice mutual pretense with those who cannot. One should take the cue from the child, telling him what he wants to know, and answering questions on his level. The child then has the freedom to speak, on his own terms, with whom and at the time he chooses. Terminally ill children may not always wish to speak of death, for they are concerned not only with dying but with living, and like the adult who is terminally ill, they wish to live as fully as possible.

Siblings are frequently neglected, not without guilt, by the parents. If their brother or sister is hospitalized, they may be prohibited from visiting. Also, they may not receive much information. Siblings, depending upon their age, should be included in family discussions about the diagnosis and prognosis. Very young children need to know that their sibling is ill and will be given medications and treatments to help him get better. Older children require more detail—the name of the disease, the kinds of treatment their sibling will receive, and possible side effects. All siblings should be warned about physical changes in the ill brother or sister, like hair loss due to chemotherapy, and weight gain or loss, especially if they have not seen their sibling during hospitalization. When the child is cared for at home, siblings can participate in care; when the child is hospitalized for a long time, the siblings are likely to grow apart.

It is difficult to avoid sibling resentment completely. So much of parents' time and energy go to the ill child that there is little left for the other children. However, even young children can understand the situation when it is explained to them, and they are more likely to accept the ill sibling and his condition when they are included in his care. Children interviewed after the death of a sibling had less resentment when they had been informed of their brother's or sister's diagnosis and told of any changes.[5] The terminally ill child also prefers that siblings be informed. One teen-ager with cancer said: "One thing I really regret is that nobody told my little sister what was going on. She was only eleven at the time. She was really scared. With little kids, they imagine things bad based on what you tell them. She's still kind of mad because nobody told her. . . . It made her scared. And nobody would tell her. In fact, I think I'm the first one who told her."[6]

## The Needs of the Terminally Ill Child

What are some of the needs of the terminally ill child? There is a need to communicate openly and truthfully with those the child is closest to, his family. The child, of any age, also needs to be able to ask questions and receive answers from his parents and physician, and to know that they are willing to discuss the illness and the topic of death. When a child is allowed to feel comfortable about asking questions, he/she will ask those that are most important, and when satisfied with the information, will feel more assured. It may take a while for the child to feel secure enough to ask these questions, but the opportunity must be there and the child needs to be aware of this.

It is helpful, when explaining the illness to the child, to draw from the child's own experience. To ensure that the issue has not become more complicated by explanation, it is advisable to ask the child to explain back what he has been told. Then parents and physician have an opportunity to correct any misconceptions that might be confusing or frightening. How the child is told is as important as what he is told, and the implications of love, concern, and hope are very important; the child may be more impressed with the how than the why. Also, as discussed in earlier chapters, there is never a time when nothing more can be done for the patient.

Like his adult counterpart, the terminally ill child needs to be able to trust his physician to inform him about his condition, to answer questions, and to educate him about treatments and side effects. All children, of any age, deserve to have unfamiliar procedures explained to them, and older children especially wish to have information about the medications they are taking and the effects of their disease. Adolescents are notably resentful of discussions that take place without them. All children, though, are suspicious when conferences take place behind closed doors, and as we have seen, they are able to surmise their prognosis without verbal communication. Patients of any age know that medical procedures are less frightening with information and advance notice, and belief in the physician's honesty contributes to the patient's peace of mind. It also allows one to feel more control in an unpredictable situation. In the words of teen-agers with cancer:

I always resented it when my doctors asked my parents to step out in the hall with them to talk about my case.

The doctor should tell the patient straight out what he's going to have to go through, unless the patient doesn't want to know. You're the one making the decisions.

The doctor won't tell me anything. He'll tell Mother, but he won't tell me. And I'm sixteen.

I think the meanest thing a doctor could do is not tell a patient. The doctors never told me what the consequences of leukemia are. They only told my mother. When I took myself off chemotherapy, my mom told me the consequences. I was shocked. She said I had five years to live. When I found that out, I was mad at the doctors; because the way I see it, it's my life and they should tell me. I should be ready for death. I'm not scared of it.

When a doctor makes you feel like he's in no hurry, and sits on the bed and asks you what you want to talk about, you really feel like that doctor cares about you.[7]

Children as well as adults need to feel that the doctor respects them as a person, will answer questions honestly, and will continue as their physician throughout the illness. After ten years of work with hospice patients, I treat child and adult patients the same. The only difference is that the child in me comes out more when I talk with a child; otherwise I find that we talk about many of the same things. Children with terminal illness often show a remarkable maturity and philosophical calm. Once, while talking with a five-year-old patient who had less than a month to live, I asked if he was angry or sad to be dying. With the wisdom of a sage, the little boy gave a beautiful reply: "Well, you know, Dr. Buckingham, nothing is forever."

Another little boy, an unofficial patient of mine, was able to die at home surrounded with love, as both child and parents had wanted. Billy was four years old and in the last phase of leukemia. Without special arrangements, he would have died in the hospital, like most other children with his disease, for there was no hospice program for children at the time and the hospital did not have a home-care service. However, the hospice I worked with set up a consultant program for the family, with the cooperation of the child's physician, a social worker from another agency, and clergymen from the Yale School of Divinity.

Little Billy sensed his approaching death and wanted his parents' attention most of all. Every night he asked to sleep with his parents, and frail as he was, his parents took him into bed with them. The little boy would lie between them, as both parents held him gently through the night. He died peacefully one night, lying in bed with his mother and father. Billy's mother was holding him tenderly and knew when his heart stopped. Sad as it was to lose Billy, both parents were grateful his death had been at home, as he lay peacefully between them. Caring for Billy brought his parents closer together.

The social worker continued to meet with the family, and several of us continued to have contact with the parents. Billy had been an only child, but two years after his death he had a little sister.

The terminally ill, of any age, want to live out their lives to the fullest, whether it be ten months or ten days. When death is an accepted reality, and we are no longer anxious about prolonging our days, we are freed to enjoy each and every day as we chose. Even a very young child with a terminal illness can enjoy his life as fully as possible, and can give and receive love until the moment of separation.

The terminally ill child has many of the same needs at the end of life as the adult. He needs an open relationship with the physician, and the freedom to make choices and have some control over his situation. The choices might be about what to eat and when, the selection of visitors or activities, and the medical situation. While the adult usually has control over medical decisions, most children are dependent upon their parents. Yet if we acknowledge the wisdom of a terminally ill child, we will also listen when he/ she recognizes the end of productive aggressive treatment. The director of a children's hospice program said: "Older children sometimes ask to be left alone"—without further treatment.

In most cases, when all medical and scientific means have failed and the child is aware that he is not getting better, the children ask that treatment be discontinued and they be allowed to go home. Very young children may communicate this through their drawings or some other means. It is not just the discomfort of treatment that prompts their request, but an inner knowledge that further efforts will not cure them. Many parents have reported instances of this. The little girl whose "owie" (tumor) began to grow again after a remission wanted to discontinue treatment. Older children who have earlier been cooperative become resistant to further treatment, and wish to live out their lives in an environment of love and comfort, which respects their worth and dignity.

A child may have some desires and thoughts about how he lives his last days. Perhaps there are things he would like to say to special people, or gifts he would like to give. His parents can support and protect their child's right to make these choices and requests. Some older children and teens may wish to make out a "will," giving away some of their possessions or having their parents purchase gifts for special people. One twelve-year-old gave his small savings to his brother, "cause I don't need it now." Some children write—or dictate, if they are too weak—thank-you notes to those who helped them during their illness. Teen-agers may plan their own funerals: the music they wish played, perhaps favorite readings, the clothes they wish to be dressed in. Children of varying ages may have lots of "business" to conduct before they feel that "everything's done," and they are shown respect when allowed to do so.

Children usually wish to prepare their families. Perhaps we forget how much children love their parents, and it is tempting to fill these pages with quotes of demonstration. Children know that their death will grieve their parents and are anxious to reassure them. We hear the same message from children of all ages, from the three-year-old who comforted her big sister with, "It'll be all right," to the twelve-year-old boy who said, "I want everyone I love to understand that I'm happy and will be happy," to the teen-ager who said, "I know I'll fight as long as I can, but when I know the time has come, there's nothing more I can do, I want everyone to know it's okay. I'm worried most about my mother."[8] These children do not mind when those they love cry, for then they know that person understands and can be comforted. Some of these dying children will say, "It's okay to cry." They know they are loved and feel more comfortable with expressions of feeling.

Terminally ill children have many of the same needs as adults, though they may be expressed differently and with different effects on their families. Like adults, children need to conclude their life's business with dignity. They need respect for their worth as a person, and to die with dignity, in love and comfort. They, too, have emotional and spiritual needs which can be met. Parent and child must be the unit of care, for some of the pain of separation can be eased by closeness. Many physicians are supportive of honesty between parent and child, and encourage frankness. The health-care team (which is the norm for hospice) can help these families achieve a richness of communication, often without words. These parents and their children have little time left together, and sharing the experience of dying can be growth-filled for both. This is a time also for helping the child face death with peace and acceptance, without fear (though it's usually the child who helps his parents to do this). The parent can help himself and the child achieve a philosophical or spiritual attitude to ease the pain of their separation. This closeness is treasured, and parents who are open with their children, and are willing to discuss any topic with their dying child, feel fewer regrets later.

Donna and her mother developed a very close relationship, of open communication and discussion, throughout Donna's illness. Donna became ill with leukemia when she was fifteen, and during the next few years she and her mother became close friends, were more like two girl friends than mother and daughter. The mother was a strong woman, able to face her daughter's illness, and constantly came up with creative ideas for things Donna would enjoy—a trip, a visit to a relative, a project at home.

Donna's illness spanned five years, with many remissions and relapses. The whole family—parents, two younger brothers, and two younger sisters—were affected. Donna was most concerned about her father, who became aloof and absent during her illness. She wanted to be able to talk to him openly and feel closer to him. However, she understood his distance and knew he had trouble accepting her illness. Donna loved her parents very much and felt that her illness had brought them closer together. "Kids my age don't take the time to get into the heads of their parents," she said.

During my visits to the family, I saw the closeness Donna and her mother shared, her father's reserve, and the "normal" interaction with her brothers and sisters. All of the children in this close, upper-middle-class Catholic family understood Donna's illness to some degree. The youngest was not aware until close to the end of Donna's life of the serious nature of the disease. Donna reported that this young sister began asking her questions which showed that she realized Donna was gravely ill.

Donna had been an active girl, and was not sick until she developed leukemia. She was not told of the nature of her disease until she was sixteen and a half, a year and a half after she became ill. She did not resent this, and stated firmly that her parents had done the right thing. She felt that she couldn't have handled the information when she was fifteen. She had also been a pretty, popular girl with many friends. Toward the end of her life she saw few people besides medical staff and her family. Her friends had all left for college, so her main companion was her mother.

When I first began to work with Donna, my goal was to help her accept her short life. I quickly found that she'd already achieved acceptance. My role became that of a friend, someone she could talk to freely, outside of family and doctors and nurses. At first I saw her once a week, but soon I visited whenever I could.

Donna's life alternated between the hospital and the home.

She'd had so many remissions that doctor and family continued to hope for another, and Donna received chemotherapy until the end of her life. As much as possible, though, her care was at home. Even when hospitalized for treatment, Donna went home for weekends.

Having accepted her condition, Donna was not concerned with the future, but only with today, and focused her energy and attention on the present. She had a personal and strong relationship with God, which was the reason, she felt, that she had lived for five years. She talked to God and read prayers aloud at least twice a day, which was an important part of her life. Her spiritual life had not become active until she had leukemia. Donna maintained her faith and devotion, whether at home or in the hospital, until she died.

I knew that her parents would need bereavement follow-up. Donna had been worried about her father, and rightly so, for he had difficulty accepting her death. The mother needed support also, for Donna had been a constant companion and friend for five years. Since Donna was not a hospice patient, I requested the hospital social worker to follow up, making a bereavement visit in three weeks, after the tumult of funeral and visiting relatives had subsided.

## Home Care

Since the establishment of the modern medical center, hospitals have cared for children with cancer, including those who are terminally ill. Yet when there is no chance of the cancer being controlled, or no hope of cure in the case of a child with a disease such as cystic fibrosis, the benefits of continued hospital care are questionable. Though hospitals can provide the best possible medical treatment, can prolong life and resuscitate the dying, terminally ill people today are rejecting this setting in favor of dying in quieter surroundings, with peace and dignity.

Though the young have had the least opportunity to fulfill that desire, the trend today toward alternatives to hospital care for the terminally ill has extended to children, for whom this usually means home care. More and more advantages are being found in the quality of care received and the psychological benefits for the family.

Despite hospitals' efforts to accommodate children's needs, in more cheerfully decorated surroundings and more generous visiting privileges for parents, the setting is still upsetting to most children. Children of grade school age and younger react most strongly to changes in their environment and may have a hard time believing that the hospital is for their benefit. They may feel punished by hospitalization, as if their parents are sending them away.

The child may get to know and feel comfortable with some staff members in a hospital, but staff continuity is not the norm. Instead the child may receive visits from several different physicians, often several together, so that it is very difficult to establish a relationship with any of them. The young patient may feel isolated and alone. The teen-aged patients quoted on previous pages keenly disliked the lack of privacy in hospitals as well as hospital food, and described being treated as an object to be "gawked" at. Also, the hospital has been the setting for many painful treatments, and it is hard for a child not to feel anxious whenever a new staff member enters the room. The patient will wonder what new unpleasantness is in store for him. Will he be "stuck" again?

As was discussed earlier, death can be seen as failure in the acute-care setting, and it is tempting to use resuscitation equipment. This can needlessly prolong a child's suffering as well as the anxiety of the parents.

Terminally ill children need an abundance of affection, which is given more naturally in the home. At home, the child has the comfort and security of familiar surroundings, and the family life around him can be very reassuring. Some dying children like to be in the midst of this activity and prefer to have their bed in the family room or on the living room couch. At home, too, they can eat the food they like and are used to, and have the company of brothers and sisters and pets, and the loving care of parents and grandparents.

Home care is more satisfying for the parents and the rest of the family as well. When the child is in the hospital, all family members feel the stress. Parents feel helpless to prevent their child's suffering, or to care for him/her. In the hospital, nurses and doctors care for the child while the parent stands helplessly by. There is little a parent can do without staff permission.

At home, parents have unlimited access to their child and are the primary care givers. As less time is taken traveling from home to hospital, the parents' energy can be used more constructively for the child. One parent may choose to become the primary care giver while the other parent works; or both parents may choose part-time work, depending upon the financial situation. Usually, though, the mother remains home while the father continues to work full-time. Both, though, need to participate and share in caring for the child, and both need occasional relief from this task. Optimally, the parents work out some arrangement to share the care, feeling close to the child and giving each other some respite. The employed parent might care for the child on weekends. Family life is more "normal" with the terminally ill child at home, but even with the help of brothers, sisters, relatives, and friends, the task is arduous, requiring the support of a health-care team.

As few hospices were offering care for children at the time, the National Cancer Institute (NCI) funded a project to study the feasibility of home care for dying children in 1976. Dr. Ida Martinson was project director and utilized many hospice-like concepts. They included a nursing team of a primary nurse and back-up nurse (providing twenty-four-hour, on-call support, seven days a week); the training of a primary care person in the home (usually the mother); home visits by the child's physician and a nurse when needed; the child's comfort viewed as the main concern; and emotional support for the parents by the nurse throughout the care and following death. Communication between team members was crucial, as well as promptness in responding to the family's needs. Problems sometimes develop quickly at home, and when the home-care nurse responded promptly, it often made the difference between continued care at home or rehospitalization. The child's suffering was quickly attended to, to the relief of the whole family. Home-care nurses often carried "beepers," which added to the security and peace of mind of the primary-care person.

Pain control was of major importance in the success of this project. The nurse had to be knowledgeable about pain control as well as aware of the child's changing needs. If the child's physician prescribed a range of doses of analgesics, which could be altered depending upon the child's needs, the nurse and parents were better able to control pain. It was helpful to have more powerful analgesics available, if necessary. Given these conditions, pain could be controlled as well at home as in the hospital, and it was important that both child and parents understood this.[9] Over a period of a year, twenty-seven children died at home and five reentered the hospital shortly before death. Two of them entered for pain control and died within a day; in both cases, medications were given in the hospital which had been available to other children at home. If stronger analgesics had been available to these children at home, they would not have died in the hospital.

Sometimes, as noted previously, patients (or their parents) as well as health-care professionals are reluctant to use potentially addictive drugs, or are afraid that these drugs would not be effective later if needed. However, comfort is paramount for these children, and pain control can make a vital difference for them, ensuring a peaceful death and thereby relieving the parents. One must remember that these children do not live long enough to develop an addiction, and that they clearly need relief from pain. There is no reason for a terminally ill child to suffer with pain when analgesics are available. Dr. Martinson found that the nurse, parents, and child had to learn about preventive pain management.[10] Concepts such as these are basic to hospice care.

In the NCI project, nurses suggested other comfort measures, instructed the parents in any unfamiliar techniques they could undertake, and performed special services the parents could not do (such as catheterization), but the parents assumed direct care. The nurse was an adviser, obtained supplies, acted as an advocate in procuring analgesics for the child, and became a friend who gave emotional support to the family. Nurses, though, were careful not to interfere with the parents' care.

Nurses stayed in contact with the families following the death and attended the funeral. Parents greatly appreciated this continued support and also expressed gratitude that their child had been able to die peacefully at home. The death of a child is such an intense, personal experience that families appreciated the privacy of their own homes. Also, the care the parents were able to give their child, and the peace of the child's death, were a source of great consolation. One father expressed it beautifully: "Seth died as we had often hoped he could—cuddled in our arms before a blazing fire, in utter quiet and peace. We have such good feelings about the peace of that moment that it has been immeasurably easier to deal with this reality. We can hardly thank you and [the nurse] enough for permitting us the peace and dignity of that moment."[11]

With coordination with the medical community, home care is possible and can be done effectively. Siblings who have been included in discussions and care during the course of the child's illness can also learn from the dying child. Older dying children know that they will never get well and rarely resist to the end; in fact, they may feel acceptance and peace before the rest of the family. Though a sad time, the approach of death is also a time when love and closeness can be exchanged. The child can relax in an atmosphere of trust and give and receive messages nonverbally. He may still enjoy physical contact, a foot massage or a gentle back rub. Sometimes, especially with the dying, silence is eloquent, and the child may like the parent to sit quietly and hold his hand.

Many children thank their parents for all they have done for them, or ask forgiveness for the problems their illness has caused. The parents can take this opportunity to reassure their child and relieve the guilt he may feel. For many parents realize that painful as it has been, they've received as much from the child as they've given.

At the end, the child may withdraw attention from all but the

most important people in his life, and most children, unless coma-
tose (though some parents feel that their child continues to respond even in the coma), continue to respond to their parents. The
child may become very quiet as death approaches, yet not depressed. His energy is withdrawn from the world but he still exists,
is still with his family. He may actually feel peaceful and content.

The unspoken wish of many children is that someone loving be
with them as they die. Those who stay may find that what they
feared is no longer frightening, and that death is a peaceful,
though sad, experience. The parents will later treasure this time
and feel consolation in the thought that they and the child were
together.

A long terminal illness, and individual emotional responses and
reactions to grief, can put much strain on a marriage. When both
parents have the opportunity to care for the child together, and to
share something so meaningful as their child's death, they are less
likely to grow apart. Everyone grieves at a different rate, and at a
different time, and it is helpful if professionals prepare husbands
and wives for this.

Though there have been no studies on this, the authors know of
several single-parent families who were able to care for their terminally ill child. In these cases, the child lived with the mother,
who was able to care for her child at home. The divorced father
was also involved, to some degree, with decisionmaking and with
the child's care. One father commuted several hundred miles every weekend to help care for his son. In several instances the
father was also present at the child's death. These single parents
had great economic problems, and needed much support from
friends and families, but each one was grateful for her child's
peaceful death at home. As for the children, they expressed gratitude for the love and support of both parents.

Families, including siblings, who experienced the care and
death of their loved one at home seemed to have less difficulty
adjusting to bereavement afterward. All experienced grief, but
there were fewer regrets and less torture by guilt and doubt. Siblings had an easier time associating death with illness when the

child was cared for at home. They had a chance to say goodbye, and to finish any "business" with the deceased brother or sister.

As Ida Martinson says: "While home care may not be the best option for every child dying of cancer, it has been effective through death for over 80% of those who participated in the research project."[12]

## Hospice Programs for Children

Hospitals are still the usual site of death for terminally ill children. But as we have said, hospitals are future-oriented—that is, treatment and diagnosis have the eventual goal of cure and of returning the patient to a normal life. With the dying the future is limited, as there is no more possibility of cure, and only the present matters. For the dying child, what is important is that he/she and the family make the best use possible of the time they have left together. One mother stressed that the time she and her son had left was too precious to spend in the hospital. Though the needs of children and their families are somewhat different from the needs of terminally ill adults, it seems clear that they could benefit from the comprehensive program hospice has developed for the care of the dying. Children and their families should have the opportunity to receive complete, appropriate terminal care, a rarity in today's mammoth hospitals.

Children and their families may have even more need for hospice programs than terminally ill adults. Terminal illness is less frequent in children, and is more difficult for families to accept. The death of a child is usually a shattering experience for parents; therefore the family needs the trained emotional and psychological support that hospice is prepared to give, not only during but after the illness.

Hospice programs throughout the country that offer services for children find that the majority of parents prefer to care for their child at home, and that the family requires a good deal of support. Hospice has many advantages to offer besides twenty-four-hour availability, symptom and pain control, and emotional support (found in few hospital-based home-care programs). Hospice has trained volunteers who can provide the family with respite care or help with other siblings, and offer a variety of other supports. Hospice bereavement programs are generally excellent, and of tremendous help to bereaved parents. While some treatment centers (based in hospitals) do help families who wish home care for their child, few can offer the comprehensive program of a hospice. At one hospital treatment center, for instance, a very compassionate pediatric oncologist, a social worker, graduate student nurses, and occasional residents do make it possible for some families to provide care at home. They are willing to make home visits, to be on call, to help obtain supplies. However, they must also see to the needs of patients in the treatment center, as well as provide support for many families, and cannot be all things to all people. During a crisis it is sometimes difficult for a family at home to reach someone on the hospital team; the family also lacks the support of volunteers and the bereavement program.

The authors know of several families who cared for a child at home in a community where there was no hospice program for children. Even when doctors and nurses from the hospital cooperated, with the best of intentions, twenty-four-hour coverage was not the norm and these families endured a number of anxious times.

One family had a three-year-old dying of neuroblastoma, a cancer that develops in nerve cells and mysteriously afflicts children between infancy and five years of age. Lisa had many hospitalizations, but as much as possible her mother cared for her at home.

Lisa, like the other children we've described, knew she would die when her tumor reappeared after a remission (when her "owie" came back). The child said it had recurred before X-rays confirmed her intuition. After this Lisa did not want any further treatment. She wanted to be at home, where she was cheerful and unafraid of death. At home, she could continue her normal activities; as her mother says, "Lisa never missed *Sesame Street*, even on the day she died."

Lisa indeed died at home, in her mother's arms, cuddled in a rocking chair. Her parents were divorced, but her father was present at her death and had a chance to hold her and say goodbye. Lisa's mother recalls her death as a beautiful experience.

She recollects the hospitalizations with some bitterness, however, and has tales of insensitive doctors and nurses, questions ignored and procedures unexplained. (The mother has become an expert on her daughter's disease. As a graduate student in a related health field at the time of her child's illness, she was well able to ask questions.) Shortly after Lisa's death, she had to revisit the hospital with her older daughter. She says that the nurses avoided them and not one mentioned Lisa. She received no support after bereavement.

The experience had such a profound impact upon her that she is now a hospice volunteer, and says: "It's one of the goals of my life to help start a hospice for children." She would have appreciated hospice support while Lisa was alive and cared for at home, and bereavement follow-up after her death.

Along with the home-care program, some hospices offer another service, a day program for terminally ill children, which could fit into a working parent's schedule. This makes noninstitutional care available for a greater number of children.

Hospice programs for children serve a variety of patients with a variety of illnesses, and therefore the staffs must have a wide range of skills and knowledge of symptom control. Adult hospice patients have cancer in more than 90 percent of cases. The picture is somewhat different for children, and Hospice of Louisville reports that though half of the children they serve have cancer, a quarter of them have heart defects, heart disease, cystic fibrosis, and kidney diseases, while another quarter are neonates (newborns) and infants with birth defects. Other hospices that serve children report similar findings. The children served vary greatly in age, from neonates only a few hours old to near-adults in their late teens. Obviously the hospice staff must be adaptable, yet all programs have found that hospice concepts of care can flexibly meet many needs.

Fortunately, we are not talking of large numbers of children. Hospice of Metro Denver (which began to serve children in June

1982) anticipates about twenty-four referrals a year; about twen-
ty-nine Denver-area children died of conditions that would have
made them eligible for hospice during the preceding year. Most
other programs report about the same numbers. Yet the number
of children served may be greater than the children's hospice program figures would indicate. Some programs, such as St. Mary's
Hospice in Tucson, do not have a separate children's program, but
do serve children when needed. They find that referrals are more
likely when there is no hope of cure (as there sometimes is with
cancer), and are currently helping a child with Tay-Sachs disease
to stay at home.

Those programs which do have special services for children offered staff and volunteers in-service training in pediatric medicine
(for nurses), children's terminal illnesses, children and grief, children's perceptions of death, etc. Hospice of Metro Denver hired a
coordinator for the children's program. In many respects, however, the program is much like that offered adults. As Maureen Mor-
rell, associate director for patient care of Hospice of Louisville,
said: "The philosophy's the same." However, to implement this
philosophy her program has a separate pediatric team, with care
given by pediatric nurses. There are other additions, such as an art
therapist, to the team. "Quality time" might be different for a
child, and might mean a trip to the zoo. Children are usually
cared for at home, but the Louisville program also cares for neonates in hospitals. This highly successful program has served children from three days to seventeen years old.

One would expect that the projected need for hospice inpatient
units for children would be small, and so it has proved to be so far.
In most cases a child can be cared for at home, and the parents
will prefer this, but in some circumstances a child is better cared
for elsewhere. Environments inadequate in the care of a terminally ill child include those with many small children and families
without an adult who could perform care. Then there are abused
and battered children, and orphans. The inpatient unit could also
perform respite care, when a family is fatigued by its efforts during a long terminal illness.

These tiny inpatient units, or mini-hospices, need not have separate facilities from adult units. There is an increased community feeling when children and adults are not segregated, and there is less fragmentation of care. Children and their families will have somewhat different needs from adult patients, so it would be best if there were some special rooms for their use. Hospice aims at a "homey" environment for patients of all ages, and it is important that children be cared for in congenial surroundings. Teen-agers might need some facilities for music, perhaps stereo equipment, and since this might disturb adult patients, the music setup should be somewhat secluded, perhaps in a small lounge. There should also be a playroom for visiting siblings, which would allow for interaction between the terminally ill child and brothers and sisters. Rooms for children should be large enough to accommodate parents and grandparents, day and night. There should also be sleeping facilities, so a family may stay overnight when the child is close to death or especially needful. Many hospices with inpatient units have kitchens, for the young patients often prefer family food, and parents often wish to prepare a special treat.

The ideal hospice area for children would be specially decorated with them in mind. Children's rooms would have large windows, with interesting views (in some hospital pediatric units we have visited, the building is designed so that windows look out upon cement hospital walls). Colorful posters would decorate the walls. Rooms for older children could be made to look like comfortable dormitory rooms.

Linda Winter, a counselor at St. Mary's Hospice of Tucson, mentioned other features hospice could provide families of dying children. There could be support groups for parents (both home-care and inpatient), for siblings of dying children, and for terminally ill children. As noted earlier, children sometimes try to protect their parents, and may feel freer to express the frustrations and difficulties of a terminal illness to another child in the same situation.

A separate staff with special training in children's needs, and with special skills in communication, would not only best serve young patients, but also ensure that adults were fully attended. There would have to be enough resource people to attend to the child's emotional and spiritual needs, as well as the physical ones, and to provide the parents with abundant support. Families also benefit from guidance on the issues of autopsy and funeral planning, which requires a tactful approach.

Comprehensive programs of patient and family care already offered by hospices for adults, both at home and inpatient, can with a few alterations or additions be extended to terminally ill children. The multidisciplinary team, the attention given to patient and family, together and individually, and the home-care program so integral to hospices would be of infinite value to the dying child and his parents. Changes need not be costly, as most parents and children prefer home care. Initially, additions need only be made to increase the home-care staff. Inpatient facilities, for which the demand is smaller, could be incorporated alongside the adult unit. The physical modifications necessary for a children's unit at a hospice are minor. Rooms set aside for a playroom could also serve as a room for families who wish to stay overnight. The same could be done with a lounge area for teens.

Hospice has so much to offer terminally ill children and their families and extended families. Any life's traveler at the end of the journey, no matter at what age that journey happens to end, has a right to die with dignity, surrounded with love, and with full awareness of his/her worth as a person. The dying of all ages have much to give, and much to teach those of us on a different stage of our journey, if we allow ourselves the opportunity.

Recently, there has been an important adaptation of hospice philosophy for children to neonatal care. Neonatal intensive care units (NICUs) admit a large number of infants who will not survive, or who should not be offered life-support techniques. The emotional issues involved are very difficult for hospital staff and physicians, as well as parents. Staff is usually concerned with infant survival, and sees the death of an infant (no matter how it might develop) as a failure. There is often an insensitivity to family needs, such as a wish for some privacy with the child, a desire to hold the infant, to take pictures, and have visits from other relatives. Before the establishment of a neonatal hospice program at one hospital, "33% of families who had suffered an infant's loss in the NICU subsequently reported serious family disruption such as marital difficulty or separation."[13]

The National Hospice Program in Denver emphasizes a more sensitive, personal approach to families suffering such a loss. When the prognosis for an infant is very poor, families are advised on the option of palliative care rather than using life-sustaining technology. Palliative care, which may result in death, "can be regarded as a tragic but positive option in certain situations."[14] The decision is family-oriented, and involves a health-care team as well as the neonatologist. A family room has been created adjacent to the intensive care area of the nursery, and is furnished with equipment for the support of a critically ill infant. This quiet room, furnished with comfortable chairs, drapes, carpets, pictures, and a telephone allows the family privacy with the infant, and may be used for visits with the grandparents and other siblings, if the parents wish. The family minister may also come to baptize or to attend the infant and family. Family members are involved with the infant, though they may not be able to perform some of the nursing care.

At this Denver hospital, the entire NICU staff and volunteers were given a ten-week hospice course, with many positive results. There was an improved acceptance of death by the staff, as well as some relief in having an opportunity to discuss the difficulties in caring for these infants. As in hospice care for adults, families have participated in bereavement follow-up with great benefit. Parental appreciation has led to "an unprecedented increase in the number of letters of gratitude from families."[15] Staff morale has also improved with a new appreciation of their roles. Hospice concepts were applied with great benefit in this hospital.

## Reimbursement

We hope that every terminally ill child will be able to face death in an environment of comfort and peace; for this to happen, there will need to be more flexibility from third-party payers and other sources of funding. Earlier chapters have clearly indicated that hospice care for the terminally ill is cost effective for adults. Perhaps we can arrive at a comparable view on the cost for children from Ida Martinson's study on home care. The twenty-seven children who died at home were compared with twenty-two children who died of cancer in the hospital (1975–1976). The mean dollar cost for the hospitalized children was $443 per day. Children cared for at home had a mean daily cost of $25. Two-thirds of the cost of hospital care came from laboratory tests, while those at home had little if any laboratory tests. The use of such tests, when the diagnosis is known and the child is dying, is highly questionable. A parent whose child is dying of leukemia in a hospital cannot help but wonder why the oncologist orders these tests, which are painful and unnecessary, as the child is expected to die shortly.

Clearly, home care is less expensive and more humane for these children. Unfortunately, just as we have a tendency to fund institutional care for the elderly, so we do for children, even when it is less desirable and more costly. Again, insurance companies often reimburse aggressive treatment only, and some policies for children reimburse only for accidents. Children are not eligible for Medicare, and Medicaid is not available to them in all states. Crippled Children's Services, a state program, also varies from state to state, but generally funds hospitalization; as one mother found, she would receive help if her son was hospitalized, but not for assistance (such as a night nurse) with home care. Disabled children from a low-income family can receive SSI (Supplemental Security Income) payments, which can be used for any of the child's expenses.

Congress is presently considering legislation to fund home care for the elderly, as well as tax incentives for home care. We hope similar legislation will be forthcoming for children dying at home. We also recommend that insurance companies broaden their options to include palliative extended care for terminally ill children. Expert hospice care should indeed be available to all who are terminally ill. May the young soon have the same opportunities as adults to die with dignity, in love and comfort.

# 6 ❧
# Hospice Care for
# the Geriatric Patient

The elderly are often treated as if they had a fatal illness or an incurable disease, yet old age is rather a natural cycle of life. Aging does resemble a chronic illness in many ways, one being the loss of continuing emotional and material support. Further, aging has little hope of remission, and the eventual outcome is death.

Weisman states that many people use "senescence," the aging process, and "senility" as synonyms.[1] Senility is the result of the aging process, the impairment of old age. Some feel that like death itself, aging must be refused at all costs.

The terminally ill cancer patient and the geriatric patient share several difficulties; among them are pain, fear of death, and fear of abandonment. Combining old age and terminal illness may compound these difficulties immensely. Caring for the terminally ill aged person involves dealing with not only the cancer and its symptoms but also the special problems encountered in old age.

In this chapter, I would like to explore hospice care of the terminally ill geriatric patient and the special problems inherent in that care. I will discuss the way in which I think it is similar and how it should differ from regular hospice care. For convenience, unless otherwise stated, the term "elderly" refers to patients sixty-five years of age and older.

It is important to distinguish between the terminal stage of life and the normal process of aging. Terminal old age seems to follow a sequence similar to that of a fatal illness. However, the aging process often lasts much longer. I will discuss the care of the patient who is encountering these two processes simultaneously. Most information on aging seems to equate illness and old age. Indeed, the combination of old age and illness increases the chance of physical, social, and spiritual disabilities for the elderly. Cancer is one of the leading causes of death within the elderly population. This interaction of disease with the age of the host may be part of the reason for the increased mortality with age due to cancer.[2]

Perhaps more than any other age group, the elderly need to feel useful, cared about, respected. However, society often parallels old age with invalidism, dependence, and infirmity. If hospitals and nursing homes reflect the prejudices and assessments of society, very little is expected of the elderly, and very little may be offered them. An aged person's death is more acceptable to us in that it seems to fit into the natural order of events. Often, the death of a very old person in a hospital or nursing home is an almost casual, everyday event.

The hospice philosophy of care views death in quite a different manner. Its emphasis is on the worth and dignity of each individual and his/her life. As this philosophy is central to regular hospice care, so I think it should be central to the hospice care of the geriatric patient.

Are there any differences between the treatment of cancer in an elderly and in a younger patient? A. Exton-Smith found that elderly cancer patients experience less pain and suffering than younger cancer patients. In one of his studies, the prevalence of severe pain was 19 percent in patients seventy years and above, and 37 percent in patients under the age of seventy.[3] In less than one-quarter of elderly patients dying of cancer, moderate or severe pain is experienced. The pain is usually of relatively short duration (six and a half weeks), and can be controlled by powerful analgesics or narcotics, given at regular intervals throughout the day.[4]

As I have made clear, pain control is a primary concern of hospice care. The emphasis is on making the patient as pain-free as possible. With modern drugs and technology, it is possible to relieve most of the pain experienced by terminally ill cancer patients. The drugs should be administered regularly, and pain control can be achieved only if the patient is under constant supervision.

Though pain appears to be less insistent in elderly cancer patients, it is nonetheless present. Hospice's concern for pain control is very important for the geriatric patient, whether or not afflicted with cancer.

It is the hospice philosophy to administer drugs when they are needed, rather than wait an arbitrary time interval and risk the onset of pain. However, administering drugs to the elderly requires special care. The constrictions, among older people, of tolerance to the effect of medication is widely known. Often, dosage levels of a drug effective for a younger person prove very close to toxic for an older person, as is most often evidenced in an adverse impact on the central nervous system. Typical drugs that affect the central nervous system are tranquilizers, sedatives, antidepressants, and antihypertensants. For example, elderly people taking phenothiazine may be more susceptible to Parkinson's syndrome.[5] It is crucial that the hospice care givers be aware of these constrictions when administering drugs to the geriatric patient.

Death is a biological, psychological, spiritual, and social phenomenon. The needs of the geriatric patient are like those of any other age group. In Maslow's terms, the basic human needs are for physiological well-being, safety and security, affiliation, esteem, and self-actualization.[6] As a person ages, factors in life work against the fulfillment of these needs. In fact, old age is often characterized as a time of loss: of physical health, career, financial security, friends, family, etc. Meeting and coping with bereavement and frequent loss is one of the particular tasks of old age. Therefore, the needs of the elderly become intensified.

Though losses create a number of problems for the elderly— widowhood, decrease in self-esteem, memory failure, incontinence, isolation, dependence—what is often unique about the elderly is not the problems per se, but the fact that there are multiple problems. In addition, these multiple problems come to them at a time when the resources they possessed earlier are no longer available—financial security and emotional support among them.

What seems to be evolving here is a vicious cycle. As a person grows older, he experiences more and more losses in many aspects of his life. This intensification of basic needs comes at a time when a person's resources are low, and the cycle continues. Therefore, of everyone facing death, it is often the aged, who live the longest, who have the most difficulty in finding serene and secure circumstances in which to complete life.

I think it is important for those working at hospices to be aware of and sensitive to these losses and multiple problems of the geriatric patient. They may then be able to interweave care of the cancer patient with care of the elderly, and provide optimal care for the terminally ill geriatric patient. Although the losses and multiple problems I will discuss are ones considered to be common in old age, I think it is important to avoid making any broad generalizations. While one elderly patient may experience impaired cognitive functioning, another may not. As in any other age group, individual differences are evident and apparent.

With advancing age, many of the human physical and psychological adaptive systems operate near the end of their reserve capacity. People become more susceptible to debilitating conditions, and self-repair does not return the organism quite so near to the previous level of functioning. As a result, symptom formation comes about more readily. The onset of one illness may stimulate the onset of another. Along with the complication of illnesses, it is common for older people to have a high concern for their bodies.

In our society, old age is associated with isolation. Elderly persons often live alone, abandoned by relatives and friends. The isolated elderly, who have lost or forsaken their families and have no one to care for them, constitute the "hard core" of the social problem of old age in all countries. It is true that many families do care for the welfare of their aged family members, but a large number of families do not have the facilities, or the time and expertise, to care for their aged and/or terminally ill relatives.

The problem of isolation of the aged has implications for the hospice care of geriatric patients. I continually emphasize the concept of the patient/family as the unit of care, yet more frequently than with a younger patient, a geriatric hospice patient may not have family support. Either no family exists or they have abandoned the elderly relative. In such cases, more support from the hospice staff may be necessary; in fact, the staff may well end up as the main source of support for the geriatric patient. This support is crucial. It has been substantiated that among the aged, there is a positive association between morale and amount of contact with kin and friends. Adverse health effects are preventable with careful casework and psychological support.

Miss Atkins was an elderly patient of mine and a very independent lady. She'd worked all her life until retirement, and wanted to maintain her own way of life even during the last stages of an advanced cancer of the lung. She was in her early seventies and had no living close relatives to care for her. As the cancer spread, and she grew weaker, physicians and nurses wondered how she could fulfill her desire to stay at home.

Miss Atkins was rich in friends, however. One friend, nearly as old as she was, volunteered for part of her care. Miss Atkins also had a neighbor she'd known for many years, for both had lived on the same New England street for decades. Together, the two ladies became her primary care givers with occasional assistance by friends from church. The hospice home-care staff from Hospice, Inc., in Branford trained the two women to care for their friend. It took some coordination on the part of the home-care nurses to ensure adequate communication with each of the friends. All three ladies grew even closer together and found the caring experience very satisfying.

They helped each other spiritually as well, for as the disease progressed, Miss Atkins's courage and simplicity were revealed as she depended more and more upon God. The hospice chaplain was a valued guest, as was her own minister. Miss Atkins and her friends had enjoyed reading inspirational work, and now as one friend or the other read aloud to the dying woman, each passage became more meaningful. With the help of the hospice staff, the friends were able to discuss death together and Miss Atkins planned her own funeral.

Miss Atkins died at home, with both friends present. It was a peaceful death, and she was grateful to the last that she'd been able to remain in her own home. We were all thankful she'd been able to die as she wished.

Another problem of the aged is that of relocation. Old people often get sick, and some even die, when precipitously wrenched from a familiar environment and thrown into a new one. There has been much research done on the effect on the elderly patient of relocation to a nursing home; we may apply these results to a hospice facility. Involuntary relocation appears to have a greater negative impact on the elderly than on any other age group. One study found that the stress of involuntary relocation caused a decrease in health scores and attitudes;[7] while another discovered no statistical differences between elderly people who voluntarily relocated and other age groups.[8] A third study concluded there was no increase in the mortality rate of relocated elderly patients; it was felt that the most important factors in the elderly patient's adjustment to a nursing home were understanding of the patient's needs and appropriate assistance and services.[9] Several other studies support this statement. They emphasize the social worker's role in assessing the elderly patient's readiness to move, ability to cope with stress, etc.; after the move has been made, the need is for support, repetition, multiple stimulus cuing, etc. If indeed the key factor in an elderly patient's adjustment to a transfer is the support and aid of the care givers, I believe it is crucial that the hospice staff be ready to offer this kind of aid to the geriatric patient.

Other losses experienced by the aged involve cognitive functioning. We must remember that individual differences exist. Changes in the central nervous system and the peripheral sensory receptors may lower the total level of excitation and affect the level of activity. One of the most distinguishable features of aging persons is the tendency to slowness of behavior. Research has shown that sudden declines in mental acuity or psychomotor skills are viewed as being associated with terminal decline. Abruptness of changes is what distinguishes the terminal stage from normal age decline. It has been suggested that the more stable adult characteristics, like verbal ability, may be more indicative of survival potential than those functions known to be susceptible to age decline (e.g., psychomotor speed).[10]

Again, we must make the distinction between a fatal illness and terminal old age, and be alert to the interaction between illness and age. I think it is important for the hospice staff to avoid generalizations concerning a geriatric patient's thinking ability. Just because a patient is elderly, the care givers should not expect a decline in mental ability.

Mental illness is also an issue when working with the elderly. However, less than 10 percent of those over the age of sixty-five experience severe mental illness. The prevalence of milder forms of mental illness largely becomes a matter of arbitrary definition, referring to the degree to which the patient has lost the functions

Physical, social, and emotional losses are the most common causes of psychiatric disorders among the elderly. The high incidence of withdrawal and loneliness in the older population is well known. There is a high rate of suicide among the elderly. In the United States in 1979, there were 27,640 suicides, of which 5,113, or 18.5 percent, were people over the age of sixty-five. In most cases the elderly are as responsive to psychotherapy as are the young. Though depression is common among older people, it is not considered natural or inevitable. One study found that of the institutionalized elderly, over 50 percent suffer some type of emotional or mental disorder; half of those were functional mental disorders and the other half organic mental disorders.[11]

One type of psychiatric disorder linked to aging is called chronic brain syndrome. It is marked by a group of behavioral changes resulting from physical diseases of the brain; one such disease involves disturbances in blood circulation. Acute brain syndrome, which is irreversible, also exists.

A functional mental disorder may result from isolation, but unlike those of senile mental disorders, its effects are reversible through resocialization programs. If not compensated for in time, isolation may lead to serious and possible irreversible changes in cognition and other mental functions.

Mr. Rodriguez was a patient of mine who, when hospitalized, quickly showed a physical reaction to separation from his home environment and care.

He was sixty-eight, and like Miss Atkins, was dying of cancer of the lung. He wanted to die at home and was being cared for by his sister. She was an excellent primary care person, who cooked for him, bathed him, and gave him his medications. I would visit and we would spend hours talking about major league baseball. There were some tests he needed at the hospital and for a few days he did well there. He was soon to be discharged, when a nurse noticed that his pain seemed to be increasing. He became depressed and even moaned in his sleep. When I went to the hospital the nurse told me about his distress.

I was puzzled, for the medications were adequate in dosage and were given properly, before the onset of pain. Mr. Rodriguez was asleep when Í entered the room, and lying in the fetal position. His sleep was restless, and he was whining quietly. While I waited for him to awaken, I sat down and began to read the baseball magazine I'd brought for him. Without thinking, I began stroking his arm as I sat by his bedside reading. Surprisingly, as I stroked his arm Mr. Rodriguez stopped whining and fell into a deeper sleep.

The dying of all ages need love, and to know that someone who cares is there and will be there whenever needed. Touch can often convey the message more swiftly than words. The fear of abandonment, which may be unspoken, can lead to anxiety, depression, discomfort, and increased pain.

When Mr. Rodriguez was released and again under his sister's care, his pain was more easily controlled. He was able to die at home, with his sister's loving attention.

The spiritual need of the elderly may be great. In fact, it may be one of their few sources of support at this time. Like many younger hospice patients, geriatric hospice patients frequently want and need to talk about death and dying. Often, they are shut out by the living. The hospice philosophy of encouraging patients to discuss their illness and death fills this need and desire.

What about nursing homes and other institutions? How does the hospice differ from them? The aged in institutionalized settings have been viewed as the most powerless, voiceless, and invisible group in society. The elderly are often treated as if they were babies, with little thought given to the worth and dignity of the individual. The elderly patient may be treated as a disease, rather than as a living person. Death is regarded as an everyday event. Some families may place an elderly relative in a nursing home out of convenience rather than necessity.

In the hospice, the patient is viewed as a total person. Continuity of care is emphasized. Humanistic concern is integrated with expert medical and nursing care. As I have said elsewhere, the essence of the psychological care of the dying patient lies in the preservation of his dignity as a living, human being, not as a dying patient. The dying are not just takers; they are also givers.

I very much advocate hospice philosophy in caring for the geriatric patient. I do think that the elderly are neglected in our society, and often are not considered worthy human beings. I do not like the idea of old age as a period of loss. I also do not like the analogy, prevalent in our society today, of old age as a fatal illness. Perhaps the hospice philosophy will help in destroying this misconception.

At present, there are no hospices specifically designed to care for the terminally ill geriatric patient. As it develops, the hospice concept of care will have to be extended to incorporate the losses and multiple problems of the elderly. I think it will be important to separate the progression of terminal decline from the normal process of aging. Also, the interaction of disease (especially cancer) and old age is significant.

I believe that the hospice concept of care will easily be able to fulfill the needs and desires of those suffering not only from terminal cancer but also, simultaneously, from terminal old age. Though the problems may differ, the needs of the two conditions are basically the same. What the dying want most is relief from the indignities of their symptoms; continuous, competent medical care; and assurance that they won't be abandoned by the medical/ nursing staff, friends, and loved ones. These are needs and desires of the terminally ill of any age.

# 7 ✿
# After Death: Bereavement

After great pain, a formal feeling comes—
The Nerves sit ceremonious, like Tombs—
The stiff Heart questions was it He, that bore,
And Yesterday, or Centuries before?

The Feet, mechanical, go round—
Of Ground, or Air, or Ought—
A Wooden way
Regardless grown,
A Quartz contentment, like a stone—

This is the Hour of Lead—
Remembered, if outlived,
As Freezing persons, recollect the Snow—
First—Chill—then Stupor—then the letting go—

EMILY DICKINSON

In this chapter, I will focus on the family after a patient's death, and the grief reactions experienced in the variety of family relationships and hospice bereavement programs. Though the experience of loss and grief are common to all humanity, each age group and relationship faces different problems. Specifically, I will discuss the problems of children after the loss of a parent or sibling, and of mothers and fathers after the loss of a child; the reactions of adult sons and daughters to the loss of a parent; and the difficulties of widows and widowers. Each family member has a different loss to face, depending upon the relationship with the patient, the survivor's sex, age, and previous experience with loss, as well as preparation during the patient's illness. Hospice, as I have noted, helps with preparation for loss by freeing the patient/family to talk openly. Some hospices also help with funeral planning. Hospice addresses, too, the issue of bereavement with a program that follows family members as they go through the grief process.

## Grief Reactions in Adults

After a person has died, those who knew and loved him continue to suffer. Even if death has been anticipated for a long time, when it finally comes there is a resurgence of grief. The immediate reactions will not be limited to those of straightforward sorrow. The death may cause some initial numbness and then arouse a great turmoil of emotions leading to wide variations in behavior in different people.

Generally speaking, the closer and freer the relationship between child and parents in the early years, and the more opportunity for the child's healthy emergence as an individual and for a gradually evolving independence, the greater the adult person's eventual ability to sustain significant loss.

In a series of influential articles published in the early 1930s, Thomas D. Eliot drew attention to some experiences in bereavement and emphasized the importance of bereavement as a passage for individuals and families. He noted that among the immediate impacts of bereavement are a sense of abandonment, shock, and denial colored by guilt and sometimes anger, and accompanied by intense and persistent longing for the one who has died.

Depression, another aspect of grief, accompanies the awareness of meaningful loss. Depression precedes the mourning at times, intrudes itself between bouts of grieving, and falls away when the activity of grieving itself is in full sway. If depression remains, it is possible that the bereaved is not completing the grieving process.

Through therapy with a hospice bereavement counselor, grieving can be encouraged and depression will not become acute. It is necessary to understand what complete mourning means. A psychoanalytic description by J. Bowlby has pictured mourning, in both its overt and its hidden manifestations, as covering a series of three overlapping stages.[1] The first stage, set in motion by the news of death, is characterized by a kind of numbness and disbelief as the bereaved person attempts to deny the reality of what has occurred. A second stage involves the disorganization of the bereaved one's personality as the death is reluctantly accepted as fact. Eventually this state of disorganization should give way to a third stage, in which the personality of the bereaved undergoes reorganization. After the loss of a beloved person, the bereaved usually faces a major change in role and self-image, as from wife or husband to a single person. No longer can the bereaved see himself in relation to the one who died. In working through and accepting the loss of the old role and self-image, transformation occurs to new roles and a changed self-image.

These three stages, then, can be considered as constituting the complete process of mourning. Bowlby maintains, however, that an individual can become fixated at any point in the process: he can continue to reject the fact of death; he can remain disorganized, torn by intense emotions; or he can reach a stalemate in an early stage of reorganization that is insufficient for his effective response to the demands of living.

In addition to mental anguish, the bereaved will usually exhibit physical reactions—irregular or difficult breathing and deep sighing, tight sensations in the throat, physical exhaustion, sweating, lethargy, feelings of emptiness, decreased appetite, gastrointestinal disturbances, crying, auditory and visual hallucinations, insomnia.

Continued incapacitating grief is the commonest variation of the usual pattern of mourning. There is evidence that the people who at first do not demonstrate their grief may later show this chronic troubled state. To recognize a state of grief as being unduly prolonged, however, implies that there is a generally accepted length of mourning. In fact, the duration of sorrow varies enormously. Usually, the more severe mental pain eases after one or two or perhaps a few more weeks. Most assume that the grief will have largely abated within six months. This is by no means universal. In psychiatric practice and in everyday life, it is far from rare to meet people whose depression smolders on and on after their bereavement, blighting their lives for years.

Social changes stem from a disorganization of behavior. An important aspect of behavior disorganization is the experience of depersonalization, in which feelings of unreality, change, and strangeness may be experienced in relation to the self, the body, or the world. The sensation is very painful and is usually accompanied by a failure to perceive feelings and emotion. Behavioral changes can cause the bereaved to disregard and alienate family and friends and neglect previous daily life concerns. Unresolved grief can affect every area of an adult's life, and without help may cause suffering for years.

A mother began participating in a self-help group of bereaved parents after ten years of intense mourning and grief for a young son, her only child. During those years she'd consulted psychiatrists, but found no relief as she felt that they could not relate to her experience. After a year in the group, she was able, with the encouragement of other parents, to talk about the accident that killed her son. She had not been able to talk openly about it all those years, and had avoided anything that reminded her of the incident or of her son. Though she still has some sadness when past memories are revived—which is common—she is more relaxed and cheerful now. The tension and anger have nearly disappeared. Her relations with others have improved and she is now an active member of the group and helps newly bereaved parents. She also represents the group in public, describing her experience for classes in parental bereavement.

## Loss in Childhood

The death of a parent is potentially the most traumatic experience that can occur in childhood. Because it is such a shock, the child goes through a period of denial until he can come to terms with the reality. Even though there is an intellectual understanding of what has occurred, until there is an emotional understanding the child will be unable to continue in his emotional and psychological growth. Knowing and understanding that a loved person is dead is not the same as accepting it.

The knowledge the child has concerning the death of the parent is extremely important to his psychological well-being. He can make an easier adjustment if he is allowed to know what is happening during the various stages of his parent's death. The child who is sheltered from the experience of death somehow feels he is to blame for the death or disappearance of his parent. This can have severe repercussions later, in emotional or psychological problems. Once the child has integrated the death, it will always be part of him, but he will be able to move on to new relationships, and have fond memories of the dead parent that won't overwhelm him. Successful resolution of the mourning process implies that the deceased will remain "a living memory," without the pain that originally accompanied the grief reaction.[2]

For years it was believed that children could not handle a traumatic event such as death. They were often told that the person who had died had "gone to sleep" or on a long journey. Many of these children wondered why the individual had left without saying goodbye, and felt they had done something wrong that had caused the person to leave so suddenly. Because of these conflicting feelings, the children would suffer from guilt, from depression, and from anger at having been abandoned. The child feels deserted, he wonders what he may have done to cause the beloved one to leave him. He recalls angry feelings he once had toward the deceased or departed person, or his refusal to honor a request from that person. He believes that these thoughts or actions might, in some way, be responsible for the disappearance of the loved one.

Today, parents and psychologists alike are realizing that children do have a concept of death, and when helped, can integrate and adjust to the death of someone very close. Children are exposed to death every day of their lives. If they don't see it on television, they see it when a cat catches a bird, or when they squash a bug.

When the child learns of a death of a parent, his initial reaction is one of shock, disbelief, and denial. For him, just as for any of us, death is hard to recognize.

The child usually experiences feelings of ambivalence, unrecognized hostility, conscious and unconscious anger directed at the dead parent for leaving. For some children, tears are the beginning of relief; in others repeated and prolonged inconsolable sobbing occurs, with no sign of diminishing. Some children have such an intense sadness that it is hard for the remaining parent to console them.

With a parent's help, children can work through their grief. Parents should not be afraid to show emotion in front of their children. Instead of being harmful and upsetting, it can be helpful and comforting for the child to see that the parent is also suffering a loss. Seeing the parent composed may confuse the child, and he may wonder how something that could make him hurt so much would not affect the parent. The child might think there is something wrong with him. "It offers great support to a child in facing his own tears to see and feel his parent's ability to experience fully his own grief."[3]

To help them deal with their grief, children have several coping mechanisms. Withdrawal is one means. Customary activities or mementos may hold too much remembrance for the child to bear. To protect himself from being overwhelmed by sad feelings, the child will shy away from activities and objects that used to give him so much pleasure.

Denial is another grief reaction to the death of a parent. It is exhibited in the continuation of rituals in which the child and the deceased parent participated together. The child's immediate return to play after being informed of the death is not an indication of callousness or unconcern. It is just a form of denial. These actions are in reality a return to the familiar to allow the child time to assimilate and accept what is horrible, new, and unfamiliar.[4]

Children should be able to work through grief at their own level of emotional and cognitive maturity. They should be encouraged to express their feelings, concerns, and questions, all of which should be answered with sympathy, candor, clarity, and an invitation to ask more questions. Most important is that children be told that death is real, irreversible, and no one's fault.[5]

Remembrance and longing constitute another step in the bereavement process. Attachment to a love object is never withdrawn easily. The unavailability of the loved person calls forth longing. Through this remembrance and longing process the child is able to detach himself from the dead parent.

The child may show a certain amount of ambivalence and hostility toward the parent in his attempt to lessen the emotional impact his memories have on him. Defense mechanisms can be the greatest interference in the bereaved child's attempt to accept the fact of death, and then to continue on with life.

When the surviving parent is aware of these defenses, he can help the child to overcome them. One means could be the act of helping the child do something he used to do with the dead parent, and acknowledging the fact that it does produce a sad feeling, but one that will diminish in time. When a surviving parent cannot mourn adequately or cannot empathize with the child's feelings of loss, the child sometimes experiences the barrier as a partial loss of the living parent. "Usually when a parent dies the child loses both parents, one to death and one to mourning."[6]

If the parent dies of a long-term illness, it can have either a beneficial or a harmful effect on the child's mourning process; the difference lies in what the child was told concerning the illness, and in the child's participation in the illness. Under the right circumstances, contact with the dying can be useful to a youngster. It may diminish the mystery of death, and help develop more realistic ways of coping. It can open avenues of communication that reduce the loneliness often felt by both the living and the dying. The opportunity to bring a moment of happiness to a dying individual may help a child feel useful and less helpless.

A child taken to visit the parent in the hospital should be prepared for changes, especially if there have been drastic ones since the child last saw the parent; there should be warnings about any machinery that might be in the room. Instead of being told that the parent is going to die, which would put a strain on the time left together, the child should be informed that the doctors are doing all they can for the parent and they can't be sure about what will happen in the future. "The terminally ill patient should explain that he has no control over death, but is receiving the best care possible and will remain alive as long as possible." [7]

An honest approach to what is happening is best for the child. Later problems can be avoided if the child is allowed to participate with the rest of the family in mourning, going to the funeral, and visiting the grave. Otherwise, the sudden removal of the loved one, without explanation or concrete evidence of the death, may induce the child to imagine that he somehow caused the parent to leave, a misconception that can result in lifelong guilt. This is also true if the lost one is a sibling. Every child has had occasional angry thoughts about siblings, and if the reason for illness and death is not explained, the child may imagine his own anger to have been the cause.

If the parent or sibling dies in a hospice inpatient or home-care program, the surviving child will in all likelihood have fewer difficulties. Frequent visits, and participation in the dying person's care, help make the death more acceptable and leave the survivors with fewer regrets. It still may be difficult for the child to face the reality of loss, for even in the case of a prolonged illness the child may have entertained hopes of recovery.

When faced with the reality of their loss, some children are not able to express their feelings in socially acceptable ways, and explode in serious antisocial acts. Bottled-up distress over the death of a parent may manifest itself in resistance to normal cooperation, change in moods, minor physical symptoms such as aches and pains or inability to sleep or eat, as well as more serious symptoms, such as lying, stealing, and bed wetting. [8]

The following behavioral patterns can be a warning that psychiatric help may be needed for a bereaved child:

1. The child who appears to show no grief at all may be in trouble and have problems much later in life.
2. If a child maintains an unshakable fixation on the lost love object, if he

continues to believe that the dead person will return for more than a
week or so, he may need aid to give up his fantasy and deal with the
reality of the situation.

3. If the child ceases to function in school or turns to severe delinquent
activities (some decline in school work is to be expected, but complete
absorption in day dreams is a call for help.)

4. The child whose anger leads him to strike out at society by stealing or
other illegal and unsocial acts, also needs help.[9]

Parents should recognize the fact that in order for a child to
mourn the dead parent, he not only needs his own recollections of
that parent; he also requires the surviving parent's help in con-
firming the objective truths of his memories, of both positive and
negative aspects of the dead parent's personality. Further knowledge of the dead parent is needed in each new stage of the child's
personality development. In this way the parent is included in the
child's growing personality, and yet the child can differentiate
himself from the parent.[10]

The ambivalence a child feels at a parent's death is also present
if a sibling has died. While mourning the lost brother or sister, the
child may feel relief that the parents are no longer occupied with
caring for the terminally ill sibling. A recurring theme among
surviving siblings seems to be that the parents were so lost in their
own grief at the time that they were unable to comfort the living
children. The child may feel quite alone at this time. The child
may also wonder if he might become ill with the disease the sibling died from. It is a good idea for parents, and deceased children's doctors, to reassure surviving children that they are well
and unlikely to become ill with the same disease. If the disease was
hereditary (such as cystic fibrosis) and another sibling does have it,
it may help to point out that the disease is different in each case,
and that new treatments are being discovered all the time.

Some hospices offer support groups for siblings of terminally ill
or deceased children. Lacking them, the hospice will know of
available resources in the community. A support group of other
siblings in a similar situation can help a child resolve feelings of
loss and guilt.

In conclusion, we must remember that adults caring for a bereaved child must appreciate the limits of what can be done to alleviate the child's sadness. The surviving parent needs to accept and respect the child's feelings. The primary task is to comfort and support a child as he longs for the return of his loved one, grapples to understand the permanence of the loss, and, in his unique way, experiences the mourning process.

## Bereaved Mothers and Fathers

The loss of a child is one of the greatest sorrows an adult can face. We will discuss mothers and fathers separately, though both are parents with the same loss, for in our culture men and women grieve differently and society expects different behavior from them during mourning. Harriet Sarnoff Schiff described this experience very well in *The Bereaved Parent*. She was offered much sympathy after her son died and was allowed to cry and mourn freely, while her husband was expected to suppress all outward show of grief and to go to work as usual. Self-help groups for bereaved parents also reflect this, with mothers attending more frequently and expressing their grief more openly. Fathers are often asked, "How's your wife?" and rarely asked how they are bearing the loss. It is beyond the scope of this chapter to discuss the reasons for this, or the history of mourning customs in our culture, but one can recall movies and novels in which women weep following a death while men remain silent or subdued.

Everyone grieves at an individual pace, and these variations sometimes place a great strain upon a marriage. It is estimated that as many as 90 percent of bereaved couples have serious marital difficulties after their child's death.[11] One possible cause of this is that each parent is going through grief at a different pace and can seldom afford the psychological energy to support the other. This is another area where a hospice bereavement program can benefit many families.

The death of a child is very different from the death of parents or siblings. For a woman, having a child is a unique event. To lose a child is like losing a part of herself, which indeed she has.

The mourning process of a woman can last for months or even years. Some women mourn for a lifetime if proper intervention is not provided. Most women will go through a period of feeling dazed and depressed. They will feel numb, angry, guilty, and sometimes wish they were dead. There is a process of pining and thinking for a fleeting moment that the child is back. Sometimes the mother will actually forget and call the child, or even buy him something.

Keep in mind that parents, and especially mothers, will grieve in many different ways. The age of the child, the child's previous health, and the closeness of the relationship are all variables. It takes time for a woman to develop memories of her child.[12]

The first stage, of shock and disbelief, usually lasts a day or even longer. The numbness a woman feels is really a protection for her and allows her time to attend to immediate matters. If this state of shock and disbelief persists for several days, it is a signal that something is wrong, an indicator of unyielding grief. Other immediate effects of bereavement for the mother may be a feeling of abandonment, a rejection of the facts involving the death, accident proneness, self-blame, and/or vengefulness toward someone she blames for the death. Many times a mother will blame God or even her husband. If a marital relationship can sustain the death of a child, then the marriage is likely to be very stable. Many women will doubt their adequacy as mother or wife.[13]

During the state of longing for the child, the mother will experience waves of memories and images of her child. Memories can be triggered by a toy, a holiday, or a playmate the child had in school. This preoccupation with the dead child is actually a gradual adaptation to the loss, and is part of the grief process. During this second stage, which lasts for about a year, peaking at about three months, some of the following behavior may be observed:[14]

- Escaping from the death through drugs or alcohol, moving to a new house, social distractions, or work.
- Removing all reminders of the child, deliberately forgetting or refusing to talk about the child.
- Becoming a recluse.

- Identifying with the child.
- Reattaching affections to a new child to replace the deceased one, or constantly espousing charities or causes, usually related to the child's illness.

Most of these behavior patterns take time to develop. Some women think they must fit into a model when they are going through the bereavement process. They feel guilty if they do not follow the standard pattern of grief. But in our culture, there is no standard for death.

It is hard for a parent, especially a mother, to return to the normal way of life. She wants to talk about the loss, but her friends and family may be reluctant to listen. It is very important to let a woman express her thoughts and feelings about her child's death. If she keeps them bottled up inside, the grieving process will take much longer. Talking about painful memories and episodes of sadness will help the mother, and gradually the past will become much easier to talk about. The emptiness will remain for shorter periods and will go away for longer periods. In this way the mother is saying goodbye, bit by bit, and the pain is not so harsh. Soon, when the goodbye is complete, all the mother has left are the memories of the child, and the pain is gone. If the goodbye is never completed, the bereaved mother will never return to the world of living.

The great strain the death of a child places upon the father often goes unrelieved. Men in our society are expected to remain in control, even in times of crisis or emotional upheaval. Society's view of the traditional male role may be the basis for much misunderstanding of the grieving father. Of course, grief reactions differ from father to father, but generally, men display less emotion than women. Their denial of feelings may lead to increased use of alcohol or narcotics, severe depression, withdrawal from everyday activities, or other long-term traumatic conditions.

Interestingly, the anticipatory grief associated with the care of a terminally ill child may cause more emotional trauma for a father than for a mother. Mothers are traditionally the main care givers, while fathers are breadwinners. If the child is in a care facility, the father may visit infrequently, thus failing to accommodate himself to the problems—of the child, the mother, and the staff—that he encounters. A child may naturally be tired and irritable, the mother distressed, the staff harried. Fathers are more likely to react by withdrawing totally from the situation; they can easily resort to immersion in their work. Mothers will accept the inevitable first because they have seen more crises and welcome death as relief. It is no wonder that parents are rarely in the same stages of grief.

As death approaches, some fathers cannot stay in the room. They feel helpless and useless. They fear they will break down and lose control. The emotions that are voiced are tremendous guilt, frustration, anger, and self-hatred. Most fathers remain withdrawn and closed-mouthed. Mothers resent this and say,"He doesn't care, he isn't grieving at all."

Sometimes it is easier for a father to talk to another bereaved father about the loss, someone who has been through the experience. In fact, both parents may find it easier to talk with others who have shared a similar experience, others who know how hard it is to go on with daily living, who understand how long it takes for the ache to subside. Bereavement support groups (organized in nearly every hospice) can help a husband and wife through the grieving process, with patient understanding. Hospice bereavement programs can also make referrals for other kinds of counseling (when not offered at the hospice), such as financial advice for couples burdened with debts after a child's prolonged illness. Such burdens, when couples are already burdened with grief, can become overwhelming. Indeed, bereavement support is essential for the survival of many families.

Family members need each other's compassion and love to recover from the loss of a child. Patience and gentleness can ease the pain of grief and allow the wounds to heal.

## Parental Loss in Adulthood

Many hospice patients are older people suffering from terminal illness, who will leave grown children behind. Most adults do feel grief over the loss of a parent, including some shock and numbness. Many people observe change in their self-image following the death of a parent, and some become aware of the emergence of a part of themselves that reflects the dead parent.

As with other sorts of bereavement, there is a tendency to idealize the lost parent. Sometimes there is a negative tendency as well (remembering the dead parent as worse than he or she probably was). Those who have the most difficulty with mourning and grief are those with unfinished "business." When the survivor feels ambivalence toward the deceased, as well as some responsibility or guilt over the past, there may be more difficulty resolving the grief.

Daughters often have (or report) more difficulty with loss after the death of a parent. This may be because daughters tend to maintain closer ties with parents in adulthood, and/or because women feel less inhibited about expressing grief. Also, daughters are more likely to have attended the parent during a terminal illness. When this occurs with hospice support, there may well be fewer problems, and less unfinished business.

Daughters—and sons—who cared for a parent with hospice support, either at home or at the inpatient unit, will have received much support for anticipatory grief, and during the bereavement period will receive visits from the hospice bereavement team. In addition, friends and family, religious and philosophical beliefs, and urgent life concerns can all help the adult son or daughter to cope. Most adults see the loss of their parent as painful, but experience some beneficial growth.

The meaning of the loss of a parent is often largely internal and symbolic. The death of a parent marks the end of one's oldest relationship and affects one's relationships with survivors.

## Widows and Widowers

It has been said that when one loses a child one loses one's future, and when one loses a parent one loses one's past, but when the loss is the spouse, one seems to lose the present. Widowers and widows have so many adjustments to make that, again, the need for hospice bereavement programs is self-evident.

The psychological response to bereavement involves a period, often a year or two, of grief and mourning during which the survivor's ability to function is somewhat impaired. It does not generally involve pathological symptoms unless previous symptoms were present. There is good evidence that loss of a spouse may be followed by deterioration in physical and mental health of the survivor.[15] There appear to be increases in illness, accident, and mortality rates among spouses of the deceased, perhaps partially as results of physical exhaustion, loneliness, and grief itself.[16] Middle-aged widows have been shown to experience almost universally certain emotional problems, among them depression, anxiety, apathy, insomnia, a sense of the presence of the deceased, and difficulty in accepting the fact of loss.[17]

A study of 109 widowed persons during the first month of their bereavement found that the most common symptoms were crying, depressed feelings, difficulty in sleeping, impaired concentration, poor memory, lack of appetite and weight loss, and heavy reliance on sleeping pills and tranquilizers.[18]

During the process of bereavement, preoccupation with the image of the deceased partner and the quality of the feelings aroused by that image, to the exclusion of other feeling experiences, usually diminishes as the survivor accepts the new role and begins reorganizing his/her life. This change occurs to the extent that the widowed person is able to adopt new modes of interaction, new pastimes and relationships.

It has been determined that preparation for the loss lessens the potential for abnormal or extreme grief reactions. The duration and the nature of the illness, particularly with respect to changes in the dying individual, also appear to influence the grief reaction of the survivor, thus affecting later readjustment.

The widow who is allowed, by friends and by society, to express her thoughts and display her emotions is likely to have less difficulty working through the grief process and thus will begin her readjustment earlier. The greater the variety of socially valuable roles and functions the widow may choose from, the more she is reoriented with a sense of meaning, purpose, and productivity in life, which are essential to her identity.

Change in economic status particularly burdens a surviving woman. Loss of income may result in financial insecurity, personal anxiety, and frustration. The widow may be forced to seek employment, but often she may lack adequate employable skills. The presence of training programs or employment counselors may make a large difference in the widow's adaptation.

The social situation of the widow at the time of and following the death of her spouse affects her readjustment. Particularly important is the availability of meaningful relationships, both similar to and different from the one cut off by the loss. The cultural patterns of the widow and her society, including rituals and religious beliefs, are significant in facilitating or inhibiting mourning.

Giving up the old role of wife and seeking a new identity is very difficult. The widow must manage many unaccustomed tasks that were formerly done by her husband. In other ways, also, it is difficult to find the way to a new identity. Diane Kennedy Pike described this experience, and the transition from the dynamic relationship of a wife to feeling like a nonentity as a widow. When interviewed, or engaged to speak in public, she was invariably referred to as "the widow of James Pike" (a well-known author, speaker, and bishop), and found that people expected his views and not hers. As she says, "to be Jim's 'widow' felt restrictive—like having identity only in relation to what once was, to be wedded to the past."[19]

Most widows have considerable financial strain to adjust to. The medical bills may have exceeded insurance reimbursement during a long terminal illness. If the husband was the major wage earner, the widow may face a limited income and lowered standard of living. If there are children to raise as well, she has further considerations.

In our culture, the widow may very well be denied the support she needs. "Every widow discovers that people who were previously friendly and approachable become embarrassed and strained in her presence. Expressions of sympathy often have a hollow ring and offers are not followed up. It often happens that only those who share the grief or themselves suffered a major loss remain at hand. It is as if the widow has become tainted with death in much the same way as the funeral director."[20]

As a whole, American cultural patterns do not indicate a tolerance for expressions of bereavement. Geraldine Palmer described her own experience of bereavement as follows: "Not only did people not want to talk about my husband's death, they couldn't feel or understand my pain, my bewilderment, my abject grief. Not my parents, my brother, my friends, relatives, nor psychiatrist."[21]

Emmy Gut states that the middle-aged woman who loses her husband by death is likely to feel intense preoccupation with her own physical health, and to be plagued with fears of being physically or emotionally alone in the face of terminal illness and death. Unless the widow is encouraged to express her feelings and talk out her fears, the fears may be repressed without being resolved, thus enhancing risks for mental and physical breakdown. Talking about her loss helps the widow accept it.[22]

While widows have recently earned a place in society's attention, widowers, a somewhat rarer and quieter species, are often ignored. There is a tendency to assume that the widower must be getting along all right because we do not hear much from or about him.

In fact, studies of recently widowed men demonstrate an increase in mortality, an increased tendency toward depression, general symptoms of disturbance in sleep, appetite, and weight, greater consumption of alcohol and tranquilizers, a tendency to need and seek help for emotional problems, difficulty in making decisions, and an augmentation of acute physical symptoms.

Two separate studies have established a significant correlation between the widower's early stage of bereavement and an increase in widower mortality. One in 1963 recorded an increase in the death rate among 4,486 widowers of almost 40 percent during the first six months of bereavement.[23]

The widower's responses to bereavement can be traced in relation to important events in the bereavement process. The information provided below was taken from the Harvard Bereavement Study, which included nineteen widowers and forty-nine widows.[24]

Newly bereaved widowers responded to the impact of death with shock, anguish, and numbness. They were apt to report a feeling of "dismemberment," to feel "like both my arms were being cut off." Widowers were apt to feel "choked up" but most resisted the urge to cry or make a scene.

Pangs of grief or episodes of severe anxiety and psychological pain during which the widower strongly missed his spouse began within a few hours after the impact of bereavement and usually reached a peak during the second week.

Feelings of panic, a dry mouth, and other autonomic activity were also pronounced. Deep sighing respiration, restless but aimless hyperactivity, and difficulty in concentrating on anything but thoughts of loss were common.

Typically, the widower was control and reality oriented. He was unlikely to speak openly about his feelings. He did not seek out opportunities to share either the events related to his loss or his personal reactions to it. He was likely to feel uncomfortable with direct emotional expression and attempted to maintain control of his feelings, as it was considered a weakness to let go.

Widowers' responses to direct questioning by the Harvard Study interviewers indicated that most of them felt friends and family expected them to be strong, to hold up and not break down. One widower said that he had succeeded in suppressing his own feelings until he saw his father weeping at the funeral. After reacting to his father's outburst with shocked surprise, he realized that crying was an acceptable thing to do at a funeral. He himself also started to cry.

Some widowers expressed surprise and fear at the intensity of their emotions and imaginings after the impact of bereavement. They feared going mad when strong feelings of anger overcame them. Many reported vivid nightmares, distractability, and difficulty in remembering everyday matters. Some expressed concern over how they would be able to manage in the months to come. Many experienced guilt feelings and were likely to blame themselves for what they did or did not do in relation to the death: "I wasn't sensitive enough to her"; "I should have made things easier."

In the Harvard Bereavement Study the widower typically was intolerant of his impulse to dwell upon the past and forced himself to focus on the immediate realities of his situation. He resumed his work roles and other functions within a short period of time. Pangs of grief became less frequent and occurred usually only when triggered by a particular memento or event.

When the adjustment of widows and widowers was compared, the Harvard researchers at first reported that widowers overall seemed more adjusted. They showed less overt distress after bereavement than the women and appeared to have a much better psychological and social adjustment a year later. They had returned to work roles and previous functions sooner than the widows, and they began to date earlier.

However, a close look at the quality of the widowers' lives, including the occupational sphere, indicated a significant decrease in energy, competence, and satisfaction. At follow-up, two to four years after the death of the spouse, it was the men who were found to have taken longer to recover. Even though the widower appeared more adjusted, it did not mean that he had worked through his attachment to his former wife or the feelings stirred up since her death.

## Hospice Bereavement Programs

Hospice is the humane and sensible way to care for the terminally ill; bereavement follow-up after the patient's death is just as humane and sensible. The overwhelming evidence of the suffering and adjustments families must make after a loved one's death clearly indicate the need for ongoing care for the survivors. The hospice concept of treating the patient/family as the unit of care is not only humane but very practical socially. Grief, unassisted and unprepared for, can lead to delinquency of children, divorce, drug and alcohol abuse, and poor physical health.

Preparation for bereavement, which is usually an aspect of hospice care, includes preparing the will, discussing the funeral, and planning for the future. The patient and his family help each other face the inevitable. Furthermore, the closeness established between patient and family during a peaceful terminal phase can ease acceptance of death. Survivors are likely to feel less, if any, guilt, and to have little, if any, unfinished business.

The greatest grief may occur weeks or months after the death. Immediately following it, family and friends give much support. The funeral service itself may also focus community support on the newly bereaved. However, after the funeral most friends and relatives want to go back to their own lives, hopeful that the bereaved will recover quickly, with little help. It is during this time that bereavement brings great loneliness, and the unresolved need to talk about the loved one and the experience.

Hospice bereavement programs usually begin with a visit to the family a month after the death. The bereavement team includes a trained counselor or nurse and a highly trained volunteer. Many times the family will already be acquainted with the nurse or volunteer, through previous hospice care. Visits continue, with assessment at three, six and nine months. The needs of individual families vary, so not every family will require frequent visits. Another assessment visit is made at thirteen months, since the anniversary of the death is a painful time for most. Assessment can add to a family's stress, and is also inaccurate during a difficult time. Families are not forgotten and receive help from volunteers and the bereavement counselor. The anniversary is likely to be remembered in the support-group meeting for bereaved families, or in some other special way. Some families will be followed for up to two years, but for many the deepest grief will be over after a year.

Hospice bereavement programs may include individual counseling, besides the volunteer's visits, support groups, seminars on grief, and programs during the holidays. This last is particularly important, for holidays trigger memories of family gatherings and are often sad rather than happy times for the bereaved.

Risk factors in family members are noted during the initial bereavement visit, such things as: difficulty in expressing feelings, family discord, dependency, clinically depressed moods, weight disturbance, or any dysfunction. The mourner's past history of losses is important also, as well as any present feelings of anger, guilt, or denial. The social supports of the family are noted, as well as any chronic physical conditions. An adolescent, or a young woman with children at home, may have more difficulties, requiring attention. Strengths might be social supports, a sense of spirituality, enjoyable work, willingness to seek help, and a good coping history with previous losses.

Since usually the volunteer and the hospice home-care nurse have helped with funeral planning and attended the funeral, the family has often had previous contact with some member of the bereavement team. The team also includes the chaplain, the social worker, students, and volunteers. Hospices customarily make no charge for any bereavement service.

In the St. Mary's Hospice program in Tucson, a home visit is made for assessment by a hospice professional at one month, with telephone visits until the home visit at thirteen months. Volunteers supplement with additional home visits and note any problems that may require professional help. In addition, the support group meets once a week. Referrals are made to other groups, depending upon need. The program in Tucson also gives many seminars for bereaved families, with such topics as Grief and Loss, or Stress Reduction. Families are asked to fill out questionnaires on features of the program they've found most helpful, as well as any other suggestions for helping others to cope with loss.

There are special programs throughout the year, and the Christmas program seems especially beneficial as well as being lovely. Bereaved family members, children, friends, hospice staff, and volunteers receive a warm invitation to a Christmas pot-luck dinner. The program includes a candlelight service conducted by the hospice chaplain. Following dinner (with care provided for children) is an informal sharing of holiday experiences. Along with the invitation is sent a tactfully worded questionnaire that asks if the family has been through a holiday season since the death, what helped if they have, and if not, what plans the family has for the holiday; ideas that might help others facing the holidays after bereavement are solicited. These ideas are shared after dinner, with mutual benefit. Unfortunately, not all hospices have a program for the bereaved during holidays, though it seems very desirable. Holidays, particularly Christmas, are a trying time when a family member is missing.

Another useful feature of the St. Mary's program truly makes hospice a community resource: referrals come from all over the city for those who need bereavement counseling, whether their loved one has been murdered, or died during an accident, or committed suicide. Counseling thus is not limited to families whose loved one died of a terminal illness with hospice care. Since there is little follow-up for those who suffer the shock of a sudden death, it seems to me that the hospice bereavement program is truly needed by the community. St. Mary's Hospice also does a good deal to educate the community on loss and grief, and some of the counselors help with other groups throughout town, such as Parents Who've Lost Children, and a siblings group. These services include hospice bereavement counselors, but do not always take place in the hospice; they are open to all who have suffered these losses, not just the relatives of the terminally ill.

## Conclusion

We all face many griefs and losses throughout our lives when events do not turn out as we would like them to. The most powerful and disrupting grief occurs after the death of a loved one. The effects of grief are profound. Grief and loss affect so many other than the bereaved (society as well as the family suffers when divorce, or poor mental and physical health, follow a death) that a good hospice bereavement program not only is compassionate but is preventive medicine. Every one of us will be affected during

AFTER DEATH: BEREAVEMENT • 143

our lives by a loss through death, and it makes sense to fund
hospice bereavement programs as a community service. The hospice in Tucson is responding to the community's need for bereavement counseling, as well as education in dealing with grief, loss,
and resultant stress. Families who have been through a terminal
illness and death certainly need this service, but so do families who
have had a sudden or violent loss. Families faced with medical
expenses after a long illness are not likely to have the means to pay
for bereavement follow-up. As it seems clear that the whole community benefits from a hospice bereavement program (especially
when clients are not limited to hospice families), perhaps funds
will come from the community for this. Perhaps some day death
education, bereavement follow-up, and hospice bereavement programs will become standard. Grief cannot be eliminated, any
more than death can be eliminated, but it can be softened and
resolved with compassionate, knowledgeable care.

# 8 🌺
# The Future of Hospice Care in the United States

The proliferation of hospice services in the United States since Hospice, Inc., New Haven, began serving patients and families in 1974 has given us an opportunity to evaluate hospice care empirically and determine its efficacy in comparison to other forms of terminal care—nursing homes, convalescent centers, and hospitals. Recently, many evaluative studies have attested to the positive contributions that hospice has made to health care for the terminally ill, not only in terms of reducing tangible costs but in less tangible areas, such as psychosocial and spiritual benefits. Hospice appears to have been accepted by the primary agencies of the U.S. health-care system, since Medicare, Blue Cross and Blue Shield, and several private insurance carriers have approved reimbursement for many components of hospice care. Although some activities involved in hospice treatment are not readily reimbursed by many third-party payers (e.g., bereavement visits, spiritual counseling), the hospice approach as a whole has been accepted as a viable alternative in the treatment of the terminally ill.

Hospice-care proponents have directed their primary attention to the future role of hospice care in relation to the total U.S. health-care system. Three major considerations will shape that role: hospice care's acceptance by the general public through various public-awareness campaigns; its relationship with current institutions within the health-care and hospital industry; and its acceptance by physicians and other health-care personnel.

As we have cited, a recent study indicates that knowledge of hospice care among the general public is at best minimal. This same study indicated that once people were informed on the hospice concept, the vast majority approved of it and said they would select hospice care for themselves should the need arise. Other data suggest that people who have been part of hospice care are extremely satisfied with it in most cases. Since people respond favorably to the concept, hospice can acquire a definite share of the future health-care market, provided that the general public is informed of the hospice philosophy.

As a society, we need the opportunity to rethink and redefine our predominant views on death and dying. Especially since the post–World War II era, death has been an avoided subject. We have isolated ourselves from the reality of death by allowing institutions to care for the dying. Since people are currently realizing that technological medicine has definite limitations and even some undesirable outcomes, a favorable environment has arisen for the discussion and dissemination of the hospice philosophy of health care among members of our society. Also, the ever-increasing costs of traditional medicine are causing many to question the principle of life at any cost. Studies have shown that 80 percent of the health-care dollar is spent in the last year of life. The hospice-care philosophy offers increased emphasis on the quality of life with the result of an actual reduction in costs. Society is ready for changes in the current health-care system, which affords an opportunity for hospice-care proponents to spread their philosophy to the general public.

Another determinant of hospice's future is acceptance by and impact upon current health-care institutions. Will hospice care become a separate entity in competition with the accepted institutions? Given a predominant market economy like that of the United States, this scenario is a definite possibility. Hospice care may follow a course similar to that of other institutionalized health-care agencies and providers. As a variation on this scenario, certain concepts of hospice care could be incorporated into the practices of current institutions. However, it is preferred that hospice care remain intact and flourish as a health-care philosophy, rather than become a profit-maximizing, autonomous institution or be bastardized by other health-care organizations. Driven by public demand, the hospice philosophy should permeate the established institutions and thus change the current ideology of health care away from its emphasis on the primacy of technology.

Finally, since in our present health establishment physicians are perceived and accepted as the primary force, the future of hospice relies heavily on the collective attitudes of physicians toward the changing environment of the health-care system. Currently, acute-and chronic-care hospitals' administrators have the basic objective of attracting and keeping physicians on their staffs. Because physician training in the United States emphasizes technology, physicians expect a hospital to procure and maintain the latest in technological equipment for diagnosis and treatment. A public demand for a more humanistic and patient-centered approach to health care will change this basic relationship between the hospital (administrators) and the medical staff (physicians). The proliferation of the hospice-care philosophy will at least have a substantial impact upon the current overriding imperative on technology. Therefore, as this change in ideology develops, physicians will slowly be weaned away from the pervasive technological imperative and its ramifications, toward a more patient-centered practice emphasizing the total person.

Today's increasing respect for the nursing community and ancillary personnel will provide another catalyst for changes in the delivery of health care. Since nursing care, as a traditional art, stresses the total needs of the patient in day-to-day life and not just the immediate biophysical needs, this rising power within the U.S. health-care system will be a strong voice for changes in the current practices of physicians and administrators in their institutional roles. The hospice concept of care and the traditional philosophical role of nursing care are strongly linked and merge to provide a strong foundation for a more human-centered practice of health care for the future.

In the decades to come, hospice programs will become part of established health care. The Congressional Budget Office estimates that hospice programs will save the government about $109 million a year in hospital expenses. It currently costs the government about $19,660 under Medicare to care for a patient with terminal cancer during the last six months of life. Hundreds of thousands of Americans of Medicare age might be eligible for hospice care during the next few years. Hospice programs will be carefully watched under the new law authorizing limited hospice-care benefits to patients with Medicare.

As the scenario has unfolded in this decade, a strong foundation for the hospice-care philosophy has been attained. What then can be said about the future of the hospice-care philosophy in the next decade or for the next several decades? Hospice care could become an institutionalized, organizational entity and face the bureaucratization, stagnation, and eventual decay that inevitably befall all organizations in time. Alternatively, hospice care can remain as a philosophy of health care and permeate and revitalize an often impersonal and coldly technological, practitioner-centered health-care system.

We medical consumers, patients and potential patients, can help change the institutional, technological trend of today's health care. We can be assertive medical consumers, unafraid to ask questions. We must not be timid about going elsewhere if the answers we receive aren't satisfactory. We cannot be complacent or passive about our medical care, whether it's for ourselves, a family member, or a friend. We cannot be intimidated by the medical machine, but must help shape it to serve us. We can prevent hospice from becoming another bureaucratic institution by our support of holistic concepts and hospice philosophy. Patients and families can evaluate a hospice before choosing and note whether there is a multidisciplinary team, a medical director, bereavement follow-up, and consideration of the patient's nonphysical needs.

Many patient needs are not met by technical or scientific means but by a compassionate desire to care for the dying, a desire to help, and by common sense. The patients described in this book all exemplified the need for individual attention until death. Henry needed someone to visit and talk to him. Billy needed the close physical contact of his mother and father. Sol needed to be outdoors in his beloved rose garden. Donna needed time alone with God. Miss Atkins needed to maintain her independence. These were all important nonmedical needs, which could be accommodated by the hospice concept of care. In whatever setting, the hospice attitude of care is never inappropriate.

## Beginning a Hospice

I was asked to serve as a consultant when an interested group of citizens wished to form a hospice in the Lehigh Valley of Pennsylvania. The steps they took can serve as a model for other communities starting a hospice program.

- Formation of interest group (including health-care professionals).
- Needs assessment survey—a study to determine if the needs of the terminally ill in the community are being met. If there is a need for hospice, then the following steps can be taken.
- Formation of a board of directors (including physicians), after needs assessment indicates that a new hospice program will not compete with existing services.
- Selection of officers (including person in charge of fund raising).
- Securing private foundation seed money.
- Hiring medical and nursing personnel (part-time physician and three home-care nurses).
- Hiring of other staff (full-time executive director, part-time social worker, and consultant to train the staff and help develop the program). Addition of volunteer clergy.
- Education of physicians (physician support and education is crucial to any hospice program).
- Beginning home-care program (selecting home-care program director and employing nursing staff).
- Establishing volunteer program (hiring director of volunteers and developing a volunteer training and education program for all selected volunteers).

We must not allow institutional hospices to multiply like fast-food restaurants across the land. This concept of hospice is wrong.

I would rather see hospice philosophy permeating existing institutions. We need less bricks and mortar and more understanding and humane attitudes of care for the dying and for the sick. Though I am not advocating the spread of institutional hospices, I would like to see hospice home-care programs available to everyone. Home-care programs can exist without elaborate housing. Inpatient backup support may be necessary, but should be secondary to the home-care program. May all of us soon have a choice in the environment and setting for our deaths and some control over the manner of our exit.

# Appendix A

NATIONAL HOSPICE ORGANIZATION STATE
HEADQUARTERS, as of January 15, 1983
To find hospices in your location, write to the state office
nearest your home.

Alabama Hospice Organization
800 Montclair Rd.
Birmingham, AL 35213

Arkansas State Hospice Association
P.O. Box 725
Jonesboro, AR 72401

Colorado Hospice Coalition
P.O. Box 351
New Castle, CO 81647

Hospices of Florida
1840 N. Dixie Hwy.
Boca Raton, FL 33432

Illinois State Hospice Organization
1400 W. Park
Urbana, IL 61801

Indiana Association of Hospices
2200 Randalea Dr.
Fort Wayne, IN 46805

Iowa Hospice Organization
309 Third St., S.E.
Hampton, IA 50441

Association of Kansas Hospices
c/o Hospice, Inc., Topeka
1522 S.W. 8th St.
Topeka, KS 66606

Kentucky Association of Hospices
P.O. Box 1281
Henderson, KY 42420

Coalition of Maine Hospices
32 Thomas St.
Portland, ME 04102

Maryland State Hospice Network
c/o Sinai Hospital HC/H
2401 Belvedere
Baltimore, MD 21215

Hospice Federation of Mass., Inc.
c/o Hospice of Cambridge
35 Bigelow St.
Cambridge, MA 02139

Michigan Hospice Organization
205 W. Saginaw
Lansing, MI 48933

Minnesota Hospice Organization
c/o Metro Medical Center
900 S. 8th St.
Minneapolis, MN 55404

Missouri Hospice Organization
527 W. 39th St.
Kansas City, MO 64111

New Jersey Hospice Organization
760 Alexander Rd.
Princeton, NJ 08540

New York State Hospice Association, Inc.
2929 Main St.
Buffalo, NY 14214

Hospice of North Carolina, Inc.
800 St. Mary's St., Suite 401
Raleigh, NC 27605

Ohio Hospice Organization, Inc.
2181 Embury Park Rd.
Dayton, OH 45414

Oregon Council of Hospices
3833 S.E. Alder
Portland, OR 97214

Pennsylvania Hospice Network
P.O. Box 65
Pittsburgh, PA 17043

Utah Hospice Organization, Inc.
319 Washington Blvd.
Ogden, UT 84404

Washington Hospice Organization
c/o St. Peter's Hospital
413 N. Lily Rd.
Olympia, WA 98506

Hospice Organization of Wisconsin
2115 Chadbourne Ave.
Madison, WI 53705

**NATIONAL HEADQUARTERS**
**The National Hospice Organization**
**1901 North Fort Myer Drive, Suite 402**
**Arlington, VA 22209**
**telephone: (703) 243-5900**

# Appendix B

## Characteristics of Cancer Patients Identified

|  |  | Number | Percent |
|---|---|---|---|
| Age at diagnosis | 1–17 | 0 | 0 |
|  | 18–25 | 5 | 1.2 |
|  | 26–39 | 23 | 5.7 |
|  | 40–50 | 50 | 12.5 |
|  | 51–60 | 82 | 20.6 |
|  | 60–70 | 124 | 31.0 |
|  | 71+ | 114 | 29.0 |
| Sex | Male | 198 | 49.0 |
|  | Female | 200 | 51.0 |
| Race | White | 332 | 88.0 |
|  | Black | 47 | 12.0 |
|  | Other | 0 | 0 |
| Months between | 0–3 | 62 | 16.0 |
| initial diagnosis | 4–6 | 70 | 18.0 |
| and death | 7–12 | 83 | 21.0 |
|  | 13–24 | 81 | 20.0 |
|  | 25–48 | 60 | 15.0 |
|  | 49–60 | 16 | 4.0 |
|  | 61+ | 25 | 6.0 |

Although 398 patients were identified, some numbers do not total 398 because of omissions on certain records.

SOURCE: Charles L. Brindel and Timothy O'Hare. "Analyzing the Hospice Market," *Hospital Progress* 60 (October 1979): 55.

# Appendix C

## Life Expectancy and Cancer Statistics

Twenty-four million Americans today are aged 65 or older, and projections for the year 2000 predict a population of approximately 41 million Americans aged 65 or older. American Cancer Society statistics show that 55 million Americans will have cancer this year, with 400,000 dying from cancer per year.* A large percentage (94 percent) of hospice patients are cancer victims.

* John M. Flexner, "The Hospice Movement in North America," *Southern Medical Journal* 73 (May 1980): 631.

# Appendix D

Percentage of U.S. Population Aged 65 and Over, by State (April 1, 1980)

| State | Percent 65 Years and Over | State | Percent 65 Years and Over |
|---|---|---|---|
| United States | 11.3 | South Atlantic (*cont.*) | |
| New England | 12.3 | West Virginia | 12.2 |
| Maine | 12.5 | North Carolina | 10.3 |
| New Hampshire | 11.2 | South Carolina | 9.2 |
| Vermont | 11.4 | Georgia | 9.5 |
| Massachusetts | 12.7 | Florida | 17.3 |
| Rhode Island | 13.4 | | |
| Connecticut | 11.7 | East South Central | 11.3 |
| Middle Atlantic | 12.4 | Kentucky | 11.2 |
| New York | 12.3 | Tennessee | 11.3 |
| New Jersey | 11.7 | Alabama | 11.3 |
| Pennsylvania | 12.9 | Mississippi | 11.5 |
| East North Central | 10.8 | West South Central | 10.4 |
| Ohio | 10.8 | Arkansas | 13.7 |
| Indiana | 10.7 | Louisiana | 9.6 |
| Illinois | 11.0 | Oklahoma | 12.4 |
| Michigan | 9.9 | Texas | 9.6 |
| Wisconsin | 12.0 | | |
| West North Central | 12.8 | Mountain | 9.3 |
| Minnesota | 11.8 | Montana | 10.7 |
| Iowa | 13.3 | Idaho | 9.9 |
| Missouri | 13.2 | | |

Percentage of U.S. Population Aged 65 and Over, by State (April 1, 1980)
(*continued*)

| State | Percent 65 Years and Over | State | Percent 65 Years and Over |
|---|---|---|---|
| North Dakota | 12.3 | Wyoming | 7.9 |
| South Dakota | 13.2 | Colorado | 8.6 |
| Nebraska | 13.1 | New Mexico | 8.9 |
| Kansas | 13.0 | Arizona | 11.3 |
| South Atlantic | 11.8 | Utah | 7.5 |
| Delaware | 10.0 | Nevada | 8.2 |
| Maryland | 9.4 | | |
| District of Columbia | 11.6 | Pacific | 10.2 |
| Virginia | 9.4 | Washington | 10.4 |
| | | Oregon | 11.5 |
| | | California | 10.2 |
| | | Alaska | 2.9 |
| | | Hawaii | 7.9 |

SOURCE: U.S. Department of Commerce, Bureau of the Census, *Population Profile of the United States: 1981* (Washington, D.C.: U.S. Government Printing Office, 1982), Table 3–4.

# Appendix E

Death Rates for the Ten Leading Causes of Death, by Region (1979) (Per 100,000 Population)

| Cause of death | United States | New England | Middle Atlantic | East North Central | West North Central | South Atlantic | East South Central | West South Central | Mountain | Pacific |
|---|---|---|---|---|---|---|---|---|---|---|
| Heart diseases | 334.3 | 347.7 | 398.4 | 351.2 | 351.7 | 338.2 | 332.0 | 298.6 | 232.6 | 274.5 |
| Malignant neoplasms (cancer) | 181.9 | 203.3 | 208.9 | 179.9 | 184.3 | 186.5 | 175.2 | 163.3 | 135.9 | 168.7 |
| Cerebrovascular diseases | 80.5 | 76.0 | 74.1 | 79.8 | 93.9 | 85.5 | 100.1 | 85.4 | 57.6 | 72.9 |
| Accidents | 48.4 | 38.5 | 35.5 | 43.2 | 51.3 | 51.3 | 61.1 | 57.8 | 65.0 | 51.6 |
| Influenza and pneumonia | 26.7 | 31.7 | 28.2 | 24.5 | 33.7 | 26.2 | 27.9 | 26.9 | 23.6 | 23.0 |
| Certain diseases of early infancy | 10.1 | 7.2 | 9.4 | 10.3 | 10.0 | 11.0 | 11.6 | 12.8 | 9.7 | 8.3 |
| Diabetes mellitus | 15.5 | 16.2 | 18.9 | 17.1 | 15.0 | 15.5 | 15.5 | 14.5 | 12.0 | 11.0 |
| Arteriosclerosis | 13.3 | 13.6 | 12.3 | 14.7 | 17.4 | 11.7 | 13.2 | 13.6 | 11.4 | 12.3 |
| Bronchitis, emphysema, and asthma | 10.0 | 8.5 | 8.9 | 10.3 | 10.0 | 10.7 | 9.8 | 9.7 | 11.6 | 10.8 |
| Cirrhosis of the liver | 13.8 | 15.1 | 17.3 | 12.9 | 9.4 | 14.2 | 9.4 | 10.3 | 12.7 | 17.1 |

SOURCE: U.S. Department of Commerce, Bureau of the Census, *Statistical Abstract of the United States: 1981* (Washington, D.C.: U.S. Government Printing Office, 1981), Table 114.

# Appendix F

### A Comparison of Costs Between Home-Care Hospice, Hospital, and Skilled Nursing Home

"The total budget for the first year was approximately $190,650, or $522 per day. If these costs had been distributed among the patients for payment, a charge for patient care per day would have been made. The total patient care days generated by HOC [Hospice of Columbus (Ohio)] during the year was 2,940 (70 patients multiplied by the mean longevity of 42 days). When this total was distributed among 365 days, the result was 8.05 patient care days per day. If each of these patients had shared in the daily cost, the charge would have been $65 per day, for a total of $2,730 for the 42-day average enrollment.

"At the second level of analysis, only staff salaries were included. The salary budget was approximately $133,300, or $365 per day. Paying for staff salaries would have cost patients $45 per day in the program, totaling $1,890 for the average of 42 days.

"At the third level, the staff salaries were divided into costs for nursing and administrative staffs. Staff salaries for the nurses, including the home care nursing supervisor, were approximately $74,000, or $203 per day. The cost of nursing personnel would have cost the patient $25 per day, totaling $1,050 for the average of 42 days. Staff salaries for hospice administration was $59,300, or $162 per day. This would have cost the patient $20 per day, totaling $840 for the average of 42 days.

"These costs were examined in relation to those of hospital or nursing home care. The charge for hospital care in the community averaged $126 per day (private room), $5,292 for 42 days. Skilled care at a nursing home averaged $50 per day (private room), $2,100 for 42 days. Thus, participation in the HOC program for 42 days would have cost the patient the equivalent of approximately 22 days in the hospital. Of course, physician and medication charges would have been an additional expense in any hospital, nursing home, or hospice. The cost of care from HOC would have been $15 per day higher than the skilled care purchased from a nursing home. Care from HOC will become competitive with skilled care in a nursing home as HOC becomes more efficient with experience. As the core of trained volunteers to aid the patient and family is strengthened, the services they provide will save staff time and enable even more efficiency and lower costs."

Source: Larry Vande Creek, "A Homecare Hospice Profile: Description, Evaluation and Cost Analysis," *Journal of Family Practice* 14 (January 1982): 58.

# Appendix G

Mean Total Cost of Home and Hospital Care of
Matched Patient Pairs for Final Two Weeks of Life, by Diagnostic Site[a]

| | | Cost (in dollars)[b] | | | |
|---|---|---|---|---|---|
| | | Home | | Hospital | |
| SITE | | MEAN | SD[c] | MEAN | SD |
| Lung | 8 | 619 (355–982)[d] | 279 | 5,520 (3,333–9,575) | 2,090 |
| Intestinal | 6 | 433 (137–953) | 356 | 8,009 (4,609–11,645) | 3,296 |
| All Other | 5 | 71 (175–1,162) | 486 | 5,032 (3,756–6,930) | 1,276 |
| Mean total per diem | 19 | 586 42 | 362 | 6,180 441 | 2,599 |

[a] Two kidneys, one each of esophagus, uterus, and pharynx.
[b] Cost ratio: 10.5.
[c] SD: Standard deviation.
[d] Figures in parentheses are ranges.
SOURCE: Bernard S. Bloom and Priscilla D. Kissick, "Home and Hospice Cost of Terminal Illness," *Medical Care* 5 (May 1980): 562.

# Appendix H

Mean Total Cost of Home and Hospital Care of Matched Patient Pairs for Final Two Weeks of Life, by Expenditure Category

|  | Home | Hospital |
|---|---|---|
| Room | $ | $2,711 |
| Physician | 17 | |
| Nurse | 192 | |
| Home aide | 138 | |
| Pharmacy | 38 | 876 |
| Laboratory | 5 | 811 |
| Diagnostic X-ray | | 233 |
| Therapeutic X-ray | | 30 |
| Physical therapy | | 120 |
| Respiratory therapy | | 428 |
| Blood | | 309 |
| Supplies | 53 | 222 |
| Equipment rental | 32 | |
| Work loss (surviving family) | 78 | |
| All other | 33 | |
| Mean Total | $586 | $6,180 |

SOURCE: Bernard S. Bloom and Priscilla D. Kissick, "Home and Hospice Cost of Terminal Illness," *Medical Care* 18 (May 1980): 563.

# Appendix I

Comparison of U.S. Mortality Rates for Children 1–4 Years of Age, and 5–14 Years of Age, from the Leading Causes of Death in 1900 and 1967

| 1900 | Per 100,000 population | 1967 | Per 100,000 population |
|---|---|---|---|
| Influenza and pneumonia | 386.6 | Accidents | 32.4 |
| Diarrhea and enteritis | 303.0 | Congenital malformations | 9.7 |
| Diphtheria | 271.0 | Influenza and pneumonia | 9.2 |
| Tuberculosis (all forms) | 101.8 | Malignant neoplasms | 8.2 |
| Measles | 87.6 | Meningitis (except menin- | |
| Accidents (nonmotor vehicle) | 75.3 | gococcal and tuberculous) | 2.0 |
| Scarlet fever | 64.1 | Gastritis, enteritis, and colitis | 1.9 |
| Whooping cough | 60.0 | Bronchitis | 1.4 |
| Dysentery | 29.4 | Meningococcal infections | 1.2 |
| Nephritis | 19.5 | Homicide | 1.1 |
| | | Diseases of heart | 1.1 |

Leading causes of death for children 5–14 years of age

| 1900 | Per 100,000 population | 1967 | Per 100,000 population |
|---|---|---|---|
| Diphtheria | 69.7 | Accidents | 19.3 |
| Accidents, nonmotor vehicle | 38.3 | Malignant neoplasms | 6.6 |
| Pneumonia and influenza | 38.2 | Congenital malformations | 2.4 |
| Tuberculosis | 36.2 | Influenza and pneumonia | 1.7 |
| Diseases of the heart | 23.3 | Cardiovascular | |
| | | and renal disease | 1.1 |

Source: U.S. Public Health Service, "Facts of Life and Death," *PHS Publication #600* (Rockville, Md., 1970).

# Appendix J

## Evaluation of Hospice Care

Increasing demands for greater accountability are currently affecting the field of hospice care. Despite the emergence of a somewhat consistent philosophy of terminal care, the greatest portion of the literature on death and dying is theoretical and anecdotal. The lack of substantiating evidence in support of currently operative theories, the obvious need for better care, and the pending support of many service facilities all call for documentation, to replace the overabundance of conjecture and opinion in the field of death and dying with a solid foundation on which to base programs of action. The process of forming judgments regarding worth of a program for care of the terminally ill must use procedures designed for the collection and analysis of data that increase ability of hospice proponents to prove rather than merely claim the value and effectiveness of that program.

In order to justify hospice continuation as well as the proposed extension of the hospice concept, proof of the legitimacy and effectiveness of hospice programs is required. As investments in terms of professional training and community resources develop around the specialized area of hospice care, demand for proof of the validity of services will continue to increase. Determination of the extent to which current hospice programs are meeting the challenges they address is essential to improvement of the functioning of such programs in the presence of social and administrative limitations. Solutions to problems in caring for the terminally ill can be most effectively obtained through planned action based on existing knowledge, and gradual improvement based on the discovery and accretion of new knowledge. We must concentrate our present and future efforts on building adequate and appropriate evaluation methodologies and practices for existing and developing hospice programs.

## What Is Program Evaluation?

To the extent that judgment is involved in hospice decisionmaking, evaluation is taking place. Administrators, planners, and providers are involved in evaluational activities on a daily basis. The decision to hire or fire an employee, to expand facilities, to introduce a new product, are all evaluative decisions. What distinguishes program evaluation from day-to-day evaluative decisions is the use of the scientific method. The essence of the scientific method is the attempt to isolate causes of particular events or outcomes. If a particular hospice program appears to be associated with a beneficial effect, one must know whether the effect can really be attributable to the program operation or whether it might result from some external factor, such as better conditions at home, or a new level of comfort physically or emotionally, or any other change the patient experiences which is not attributed to hospice.

The first priority of any developing hospice program, hospice health-policy analysis, involves the drawing together and evaluation of existing research, evaluations, and information pertaining to hospices in this country and abroad. Policy analysis attempts to articulate and provide evidence for the pros and cons of alternative options or strategies facing a decisionmaker in the hospice arena. Ideally, it should be a synthesis of programmatic evaluation as well as a review of relevant nonexperimental and experimental research on specific and sensitive hospice issues.

Hospice programs in the United States should be evaluated:

To demonstrate to other groups that the hospice program is an effective health-care program.

To justify past or projected expenditures.

To determine costs.

To gain support for expansion of facilities.

To determine future objectives.

To determine program efficiency.

In summary, from the hospice administrator or planner perspective, program evaluation helps to answer basic questions about whether the program is good and whether it helps ensure accountability by administrators, staff, patients, and families. Evaluations should help keep the hospice emphasis on end results and should help promote training of staff.

A number of recently identified developments have focused much attention on hospice program evaluation. Among these are: (1) the growing involvement of federal government in hospice services with respect to financing and provision; (2) growing demands for public accountability; and (3) community involvement (financial and social) in rendering hospice services.

The reasons for evaluating a specific hospice program will differ, depending on the interested parties. The perspectives of the hospice agency, its administrator, the funding agency, public or patient groups and the evaluator are likely to differ in varying degrees about: (1) the objectives to be evaluated; (2) the types of evaluation that need to be conducted; (3) the research design that needs to be employed; (4) the relevant measures of program input, process, and impact; (5) the collection of the data; (6) the analysis of the data; and (7) the inferences drawn about the data.

## The Evaluation Process

The hospice program evaluation process can be subdivided into three basic categories. The first pertains to the exact specification of program objectives and concerns itself with the program planning stage. The second category relates to the organization of resources to carry out the hospice program. This can also be considered the program implementation stage. The third and probably most significant category is assessment of program performance, which may be called the program impact stage. The specification of objectives is the most crucial aspect of any beginning or developing organization. Every organization must have written goals and objectives or it cannot be understood, implemented, or evaluated.

The nature and content of the objectives must be carefully respectful of the overall goals of the hospice organization. Priorities must be set for the objectives of the hospice program, in harmony with the target population that it intends to serve. Each specific objective must be given a place in the hospice organization in order of importance, for each hospice program will have a multiplicity of specific program objectives. It must be understood that not all objectives can be scientifically evaluated.

## Use of the Scientific Method in the Evaluation Procedure

It is strongly recommended that use of the scientific method in performing hospice program evaluation be considered by the administration. It must be understood that use of the scientific method in performing such an evaluation requires considerable forethought as well as scrupulous attention to detail. Before an evaluation can take place, hospice program objectives must be identified and translated into measurable terms. Recognition of the problems with which the program must cope is advised, lest the exigencies of program development invalidate an ongoing, inflexible course of evaluation. A specific and sensitive data retrieval must be developed and utilized. Program activities should be profiled and standardized to facilitate measurement of changes that take place.

Measures used to monitor effectiveness of program activities should have proven reliability and validity. Where changes are detected, the possibility that they may be due to some factor other than the activity of the hospice program should be considered. Those effects attributable to the work of the program should be rated for durability and generalization. Progress in evaluation of hospice services should be made as a function of the use of the scientific method—the examination of specific program objectives and their attendant assumptions, the development of measurable criteria explicitly related to those specific objectives, and the controlled determination of the extent to which the objectives are met. These criteria characterize true evaluation research as distinct from subjective assessment or anecdotal reports, which so predominantly characterize most hospice program evaluation.

An evaluation of a hospice program should accomplish even more than discovery of whether and to what extent objectives have been met. An evaluation can pinpoint causes of specific successes and failures and aid in directing the program administrators toward formulas for success.

Practical problems of adhering to principles of research, in opposition to administrative considerations, constitute a greater challenge to execution of an evaluative study than do the rigors of those principles. Principles of research dictate that specific rather than entire programs should be measured, that methods and objectives of terminal-care programs should be clearly defined, and that control groups should be used as a basis for comparison. However, the nature of most hospice programs works against application of experimental methodology. Service personnel, although highly qualified for delivery of terminal care, usually lack training or skills necessary for evaluative research. Their collection and interpretation of data is likely to be unsophisticated and to suffer from the lack of strict scientific guidance. Furthermore, the irregularity with which scientific standards are adhered to by various staff members results in collection of unreliable data. Attempts at self-evaluation by hospice programs both incorporate problems of ill-prepared personnel and inevitably preclude objectivity. Personal bias is unavoidable when funding or reputation of one's program is at stake. In addition, the need to carry out self-evaluation as well as usual service activities prevents allocation of sufficient time, money, and personnel for planning, collection of data, and analysis. Unfortunately, administrative resistance and barriers, lack of resources, and failure to utilize findings frequently operate against objective evaluation, which is the preferable alternative to self-evaluation.

In terms of administrative relationships, even assuming the most favorable personal interactions, the program evaluation team is bound to be at odds to some degree with the medical/nursing team from start to finish. This organizational tension arises from a number of factors, including philosophical differences, competition for resources, the tremendous burden that proper evaluation places on the conduct of the program being evaluated, the special role of the evaluator, and differences in professional values.

The Donabedian model of evaluation research proposes an appealing solution to substitution of facilities and activities for achievement.* Donabedian perceives resources and effort expended as matters of importance in characterization of program, rather than assessment of program effectiveness. He has outlined a structure for evaluation that points to three components—structure, process, and outcome—as the basis of evaluation.

Measurement of outcomes allows determination of program effectiveness, and description of structure and process provides the basis for as-

---

* A. Donabedian, "Evaluating the Quality of Medical Care," *Milbank Memorial Fund Quarterly* 44 (1966): 166–203.

sumptions of causality. Program goals and objectives are the dependent variables of such an evaluation. One must be able to put the specific program objectives into testable hypotheses.

## Summary

Evaluation can be viewed as an independent check on the adequacy of hospice program planning. On the other hand, evaluation will contribute to the planning phase of program development by delineating problems, resources, and objectives, and by determining rational courses of action. True evaluation research allows determination of the extent to which stated program objectives are met through program activities.

Roos notes that it will be increasingly important in future years to fit program evaluation research strategies to the specific nature of the program under study and the types of decisions to be made.* Programs with clearly defined goals and objectives, where it is possible to obtain a high degree of knowledge, are appropriate for experimental and quasi-experimental designs. In contrast, programs that have ill-defined goals, that are in their beginning stages, and that show a low degree of obtainable knowledge are more appropriate for process-oriented evaluations.

Program evaluations, of both a process- and an outcome-oriented nature, can be expected to continue to grow. Program administrators, providers, planners, evaluation researchers, and policymakers will need to become increasingly sophisticated about the problems and issues involved in assessing social-service and health-care programs. This ranges from being better able to specify program objectives, components, and categories of evaluation, to the consideration of alternative research designs, data-collection systems, assessment of the reliability and validity of measures, appropriate choice of data analysis, and increased competence in making sure that the results of the program evaluation are useful to the decisionmakers for whom they are intended and are used by them.

There is an increased need under the hospice umbrella for training health professionals of all categories and exposing them to some basic

* N. P. Roos, "Evaluation, Quasi-experimentation, and Public Policy: Observations by a Short-term Bureaucrat," In J. Caporaso and L. L. Roos, Jr. (eds.), *Quasi-experimental Testing Theory and Evaluation Policy* (Chicago: Northwestern University Press, 1973).

considerations involved in the evaluation of hospice programs. Hospice health-care professionals will need to have a common understanding of the basic issues in assessing programs and be able to speak a common language. As hospice personnel participate in evaluation activities, hospice health-care professionals may learn more about themselves as well as the hospice program. Such self-discovery can contribute to increased personal and professional growth.

# Notes

## Introduction

1. R. F. Rizzo, "Hospice: Comprehensive Terminal Care," *New York State Journal of Medicine*, October 1978, p. 1902.

2. H. J. Wald, "A Hospice for Terminally Ill Patients" (Master's thesis, Columbia University, School of Architecture, 1971), pp. 12–13.

3. Sylvia Lack and Robert W. Buckingham, *First American Hospice: Three Years of Home Care* (New Haven, Conn.: 1978), p. 4.

4. Ibid., p. 5.

5. John Hinton, *Dying* (London: Hunt Barnard Printing, 1972), p. 11.

6. Sandol Stoddard, *The Hospice Movement* (New York: Stein and Day, 1978), p. 91.

7. Ibid., p. 48.

8. Ibid.

9. J. Craven and F. S. Wald, "Hospice Care for Dying Patients," *American Journal of Nursing*, October 1975, p. 1820.

10. Stoddard, p. 36.

11. Herman Feifel, *New Meanings of Death* (New York: McGraw-Hill, 1977), p. 159.

## Chapter 1: Hospice History and Philosophy

1. Stoddard, p. 28.

2. Ibid., p. 40.

3. Feifel, p. 160.

4. Ibid., p. 161.

5. Lack and Buckingham, p. 87.

6. Robert Buckingham and Dale Lupu, "A Comparative Study of Hospice Services in the United States," *American Journal of Public Health* 72 (May 1982): 455.

7. Erica Janzen, "Relief of Pain," *Nursing Forum* 13 (1974).

8. R. Lamerton, *Care of the Dying* (London: Priority Press, 1973).

9. R. Lamerton, "Care of the Dying: Pt. IV, the Pains of Death," *Nursing Times* 69 (January 1973).

10. C. M. Saunders, "The Care of the Terminal Stages of Cancer," *Annals of the Royal College of Surgeons*, Supplement to vol. 41 (1967).

11. D. L. Rabin and L. H. Rabin, "Consequences of Death for Physicians, Nurses and Hospitals," in Brim et. al., *The Dying Patient* (New York: Russell Sage, 1970).

12. R. W. Buckingham et al., "Living with the Dying: Use of the Technique of Participant Observation," *Canadian Medical Association Journal* 115, (Dec. 18, 1976), p. 1215.

13. A. Hackett and M. Weisman, "Reactions to the Imminence of Death," in Grosser, ed., *The Threat of Impending Disaster* (Cambridge, Mass.: MIT Press, 1964).

14. R. G. Twycross, "Clinical Experience with Diamorphine in Advanced Malignant Disease," *International Journal of Clinical Pharmacology, Therapy and Toxicology* 9 (1974).

15. B. M. Mount, "Use of the Brompton Mixture in Treating the Chronic Pain of Malignant Disease," *Canadian Medical Association Journal* 115 (July 17, 1976): 122–24.

16. L. LeShan, "The World of the Patient in Severe Pain of Long Duration," *Journal of Chronic Disease* 17 (1974).

17. R. Melzack, *The Puzzle of Pain* (Haimondsworth, Eng.: Penguin, 1973), p. 142.

18. Mount, op. cit.

19. Glen W. Davidson, *The Hospice: Development and Administration* (Washington, D.C.: Hemisphere Publishing Corp., 1978), p. 47.

20. Stoddard, p. 140.

21. David Shephard, "Terminal Care: Towards an Ideal," *Canadian Medical Association Journal* 115 (July 1976): 97–8.

22. Elisabeth Kübler-Ross, *On Death and Dying* (New York: Macmillan, 1969), p. 9.

23. H. Feifel, "Perception of Death," *Annals of the New York Academy of Science* 164 (1969): p. 669.
24. Stoddard, pp. 141–42.
25. Dewi W. Rees and Sylvia G. Lutkins, "Mortality of Bereavement," *British Medical Journal*, October 1967.

**Chapter 2: Types of Hospice Care**

1. Ida Marie Martinson, *Home Care for the Dying Child* (New York: Appleton-Century-Crofts, 1976), p. 9.
3. Davidson, p. 49.
4. Colin Murray Parkes, *Bereavement: Studies of Grief in Adult Life* (New York: International Universities Press, 1972), p. 131.
5. Ibid., p. 139.
6. Buckingham and Lupu, p. 460.
7. Michael Hamilton and Helen Reid, *A Hospice Handbook: A New Way to Care for the Dying* (Grand Rapids: William B. Ferdmans, 1980), p. 140.

**Chapter 3: Hospice Issues and Problems, Development and Administration**

1. Neal, White, and Buell, *Conceptualizing Quality Terminal Care for the Elderly* (Portland, Ore.: Institute on Aging, Portland State University, 1981).
2. Stoddard, p. 194.
3. Ibid., p. 195.
4. Buckingham and Lupu, p. 457.
5. "How America Treats the Elderly," *Newsweek*, Nov. 1, 1982, p. 65.
6. Stoddard, p. 182.
7. Ibid., p. 167.

**Chapter 4: Costs of Hospice Care**

1. Charles L. Breindel and Timothy O'Hare, "Analyzing the Hospice Market," *Hospital Progress* 60 (October 1979): 55.
2. LaVerne E. Perrallaz and Margaret Mollica, "Public Knowledge of Hospice Care," *Nursing Outlook* 29 (January 1981): 47.
3. Ibid., pp. 47–48.
4. William M. Markel and Virginia B. Sinon, *The Hospice Concept* (New York: American Cancer Society, 1978).
5. Larry Vande Creek, "A Homecare Hospice Profile: Description,

Evaluation and Cost Analysis," *Journal of Family Practice* 14 (January 1982): 58.

6. Anthony Amado, Beatrice A. Cronk, and Rich Mileo, "Cost of Terminal Care: Home Hospice vs. Hospital," *Nursing Outlook* 27 (August 1979); 525.

7. Bernard S. Bloom and Priscilla D. Kissick, "Home and Hospice Cost of Terminal Illness," *Medical Care* 18 (May 1980): 563.

8. Neil Hollander and David Ehrenfried, "Reimbursing Hospice Care: A Blue Cross and Blue Shield Perspective," *Hospital Progress* 60 (March 1979): 56.

9. Ibid., pp. 54–56.

10. Irene L. Beland and Joyce Passos, *Clinical Nursing*, 3d ed. (New York: Macmillan, 1975).

**Chapter 5: Hospice Programs and Dying Children**

1. Susan Schiefelbein, "Children and Cancer: New Hope for Survival," *Saturday Review*, Apr. 14, 1979, pp. 11–12.

2. "Study of Childhood Cancer's Impact on Families, Part II," *The Candlelighters Foundation Quarterly Newsletter* 2 (Spring 1982): 4.

3. "The Art of Children with Cancer: Saying What Words Can't," *The Candlelighters Foundation Quarterly Newsletter*, p. 3.

4. Ibid.

5. *Siblings of Children with Cancer* (Tucson: Biomedical Communications, University of Arizona Health Sciences Center, 1980).

6. Edith Pendleton, *Too Old to Cry . . . Too Young to Die* (Nashville: Thomas Nelson Publishers, 1980), p. 44.

7. Ibid., pp. 115–16.

8. Ibid., p. 165.

9. Ida Martinson et al., "When the Patient Is Dying: Home Care for the Child," *American Journal of Nursing*, November 1977, p. 1816.

10. Ida Martinson et al., "Facilitating Home Care for Children Dying of Cancer," *Cancer Nursing* 1 (February 1978): 44.

11. Martinson, "When the Patient Is Dying," p. 1815.

12. Martinson, "Facilitating Home Care," p. 45.

13. John Whitfield et al., "The Application of Hospice Concepts to Neonatal Care," *American Journal of the Disabled Child* 136 (May 1982): 422.

14. Ibid.

15. Ibid., p. 423.

## Chapter 6: Hospice Care for the Geriatric Patient

1. A. D. Weisman, *On Dying and Denying: A Psychiatric Study of Terminality* (New York: Behavioral Publications, 1972).
2. J. E. Birren, *The Psychology of Aging* (Englewood Cliffs, N.J.: Prentice-Hall, 1964).
3. A. N. Exton-Smith, "Terminal Illness in the Aged," *Lancet* 2 (1961): 305–8.
4. E. V. Cowdry, *Aging Better* (Springfield, Ill.: Charles C. Thomas, 1972).
5. H. S. Wang, "Special Diagnostic Procedures—The Evaluation of Brain Impairment," in E. W. Busse and E. Pfeiffer, eds., *Mental Illness in Later Life* (Washington, D.C.: American Psychiatric Association, 1973).
6. I. M. Hulicka, "Understanding Our Client, the Geriatric Patient," *Journal of the American Geriatrics Society* 29 (1972): 438–48.
7. R. M. Grey and J. M. Kasteler, "An Investigation of the Effects of Involuntary Relocation on the Health of Older Persons," *Sociological Symposium* 2 (1969): 49–58.
8. M. P. Lawton and S. Yaffe, "Mortality, Morbidity, and Voluntary Change of Residence by Older People," *Journal of the American Geriatrics Society* 18 (1970): 823–31.
9. E. H. Orgen and M. W. Linn, "Male Nursing Home Patients: Relocation and Mortality," *Journal of the American Geriatrics Society* 19 (1971): 229–39.
10. L. F. Jarvik and A. Falek, "Intellectual Stability and Survival in the Aged," *Journal of Gerontology* 18 (1963): 173–76.
11. E. Pfeiffer, "What to Do About Mental Disorders of the Elderly," *Modern Healthcare* 2 (1974): 57–61.

## Chapter 7: After Death: Bereavement

1. J. Bowlby, "Processes of Mourning," *International Journal of Psychoanalysis* 44 (1961): p. 317.
2. M. J. Shoor and M. H. Speed, "Delinquency as a Manifestation of the Mourning Process," *Psychiatric Quarterly* 37 (1963).
3. E. Furman, *A Child's Parent Dies* (New Haven: Yale University Press, 1974).
4. Ibid.
5. R. DeVaul, S. Zisook, and F. Faschingbauer, "Clinical Aspects of Grief and Bereavement," *Primary Care* 6.

6. J. E. Schowelter, "Parent's Death and Child Bereavement," in B. Schoenberg et al., ed., *Bereavement: Its Psychological Aspects* (New York: Columbia University Press, 1975).

7. H. D. Dunton, "The Child's Concept of Death," in B. Schoenberg, ed., *Loss and Grief: Psychological Management in Medical Practice* (New York: Columbia University Press, 1970).

8. D. Hedin, *Death as a Fact of Life* (New York: Norton, 1973).

9. Ibid. p. 156.

10. Furman.

11. Harriet Sarnoff Schiff, *The Bereaved Parent* (New York: Penguin Books, 1978), p. 84.

12. Jo-Eileen Gyulay, *The Dying Child* (New York: McGraw-Hill/Blakiston, 1978).

13. Charles E. Hollingsworth and Robert O. Pasnau, *The Family in Mourning: A Guide for Health Professionals* (New York: Grune & Stratton, 1977).

14. Earl A. Grollman, *Concerning Death: A Practical Guide for the Living* (Boston: Beacon Press, 1974).

15. C. M. Parkes, "Recent Bereavement as a Cause of Mental Illness," *British Journal of Psychiatry* 110 (1964a): 198–204.

16. Douglas C. Kimmel, *Adulthood and Aging* (New York: Wiley, 1974), p. 433.

17. C. M. Parkes, *Bereavement: Studies of Grief in Adult Life* (New York: International University Free Press, 1972).

18. Paul J. Clayton, James A. Halikes, and William Maurice, "The Bereavement of the Widowed," *Diseases of the Nervous System* 32 (1971): 597–604.

19. Diane Kennedy Pike, *Life Is Victorious! How to Grow Through Grief* (New York: Simon & Schuster, 1976), pp. 159–61.

20. Parkes, p. 8.

21. Geraldine Palmer, "Singles World," in Rae Lindsay, *Alone and Surviving* (New York: Walker, 1977).

22. Emmy Gut, "Some Aspects of Adult Mourning," *Omega* 5 (1974): 335.

23. M. Young, B. Benjamin, and C. Wallis, "Mortality of Widowers," *Lancet* 2 (1963): 454–56.

24. C. M. Parkes and R. Brown, "Health After Bereavement: A Controlled Study of Young Boston Widows and Widowers," *Psychosomatic Medicine* 34 (1972): 449–60.

# Index